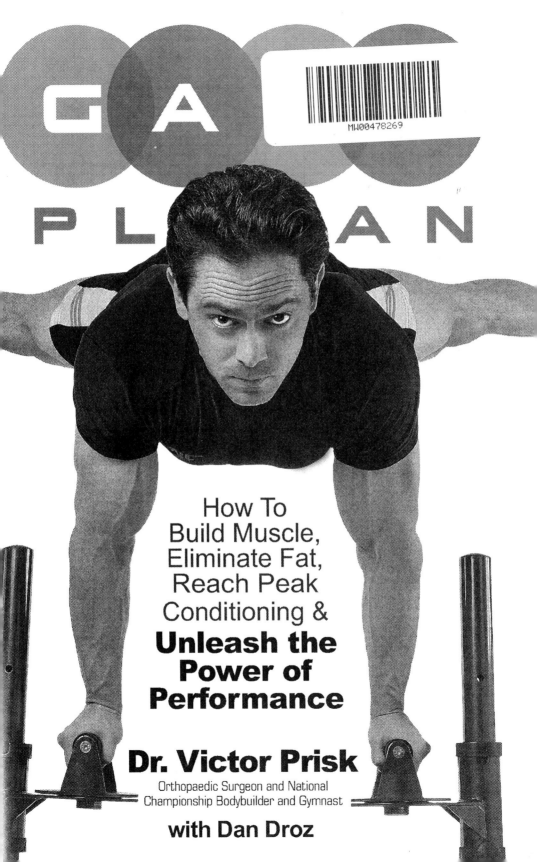

GAME PLAN

How To
Build Muscle,
Eliminate Fat,
Reach Peak
Conditioning &
**Unleash the
Power of
Performance**

Dr. Victor Prisk

Orthopaedic Surgeon and National
Championship Bodybuilder and Gymnast

with Dan Droz

Acknowledgements

I would like to thank my family, friends and the following individuals and organizations for their continued support:

- GNC
- Allegheny Health Network
- Jim Manion and the National Physique Committee (NPC)
- Steve Blechman of Advanced Research Media
- Kelly Olexa of FitFluential
- Aaron Metosky & Robert Handley of Droz Marketing

and of course, my loving wife, Dr. Kristina Curci

G.A.I.N. Plan: *How to Build Muscle, Eliminate Fat, Reach Peak Conditioning & Unleash the Power of Performance*

Published by G.A.I.N. Plan, LLC
Book Design by DROZ Marketing
Photo Credit: Alan J. King *(Front & Back Cover)*

G.A.I.N. Plan, LLC
Website: www.YourGainPlan.com

Foreward

By Kelly Olexa, *FitFluential*

I am often asked how I can explain the explosive growth of social media in the fitness and nutrition community, exemplified through the success of Victor Prisk's training and nutritional plan and *FitFluential*, the social media company I founded in 2011.

I believe that those programs like *G.A.I.N.* and *FitFluential* have succeeded because the various social media platforms where our people engage provide anyone and everyone three critical components for success.

Acceptance. Accountability. Accessibility.

What has been sorely missing for fitness enthusiasts of all kinds — at all stages of their journey is an all-inclusive community that provides them with a warm welcome and a daily opportunity to learn and discover new things without fear or intimidation.

Think about what it's like when one first decides to change their mind and body for the better. That original impetus for change is not typically a warm-fuzzy moment. Men and women often get to a point where they feel they MUST change, either due to dissatisfaction with how they look or feel or perhaps even worse, because a doctor or specialist is saying it's time to change or face some tough consequences.

As such, the start of that fitness or better health journey is often filled with intimidation, fear, uncertainty and likely a high level of discomfort. One might wonder, how do I start? Where do I look? What do I read? What's right for me?? Running?? Maybe yoga.... Crossfit?? At that point, it's easy to feel very overwhelmed and discouraged.

What were the options in the past?

What I observed — having been there myself, is that what was available in the past were limited resources, and many of them being rather EXCLUSIVE and INTIMIDATING rather than inclusive and welcoming.

Think about it. In the past, if you were considering losing weight or getting active, you might go to a Barnes & Noble or your grocery store to buy a fitness book and/or a fitness magazine. What's the problem with those options? In my opinion, while so many fitness/diet/health books are written by outstanding authors-- and the content is valid and viable...it's so often a bit too extreme. This is what sells. 12-Week transformations or workouts that are "10 Minutes a DAY!" and don't even get me started on the diet books out there. The magazines published in the fitness space assume a level of knowledge with terms and phrases that many newbies cannot relate to.

The problem isn't the books or the magazines alone. The problem is that someone can buy any great periodical or book- and still find themselves overwhelmed and confused, frustrated and alone. That's a bad place to be.

What we have seen in our *FitFluential* community and echoed in successful communities like the Dr. Prisk's *Century Club Challenge* and his *G.A.I.N. Plan*, is that the men and women that have "been there, done that" are able to connect with anyone that is a complete newbie just starting out, and immediately give them encouragement, motivation and a feeling that, hey-- you are not ALONE. These newbies can ask anything and everything-- perhaps about that 12-Week transformation book they just picked up or a diet approach they saw on TV. The intimidation factor is gone. The feeling of family and "Hey, I BELONG HERE" is turned on the second they start connecting with others. It also gives them an opportunity to share the results of their effort, whether through a few poses that show off their newly honed abs or even a great dinner prepared with just the right nutrients for a healthy diet.

It's a really cool thing to witness. One can almost HEAR a huge sigh of relief when someone who has just started gets warmly welcomed by strangers they've never met. These strangers will often become close friends with that newbie and sometimes coaches — either way, we witness strongly loyal relationships developing every day. And then, we see lives changing.

Just as there is no one way to get fit, lose weight and improve your health, there is no ONE social media platform that is the magic solution. Our people connect via blogs, YouTube channels, Facebook, Twitter, Pinterest, Instagram and more. These platforms and the 24-hour accessibility have leveled the playing field in myriad ways, and all for the better.

The social media field and ideas presented in this book are ones that embrace all kinds of sports and fitness pursuits. We have members with virtually every dietary preference or restriction on the planet. My personal goal has always been to showcase all of these-- always promoting individuals that reflect a positive inspiring attitude toward others. I absolutely love to see how all of these formerly disparate communities-- runners, crossfitters, bodybuilders, stroller stride mommies, triathletes, football players, cheerleaders, yogis and Zumba fanatics can connect with one another and often influence each other to step outside the norm and try something new.

At *FitFluential*, Our tagline is Fitness Found™.

I believe we've created a thriving community that allows everyone to do just that-- find their fitness. Fitness is no longer as cut and dry as it used to be and this is why this social media landscape in which we play allows everyone to branch out. Without the ability to connect with new friends 24/7 and learn about new sports or events or classes, perhaps men and women would more easily settle in to labels that existing years ago like "I'm a runner." or "I do yoga".

Fitness now is defined by each individual. And that is a beautiful thing. We see folks that start losing weight by walking on their lunch hour. Suddenly they discover crossfit and are changing their lives and getting their co-workers and families involved. We see figure competitors embracing something new like yoga or rock climbing to add variety to their training. We see yogis adding kettlebell training and sometimes moving into bodybuilding. There are no rules anymore and there are no limiting labels. *The G.A.I.N. Plan* is a new way to embrace these enduring principles:

ACCEPTANCE.

Everything that can be tough about getting started or getting "back on track" evaporates when you feel INCLUDED. When you know that you are not alone, you feel inspired and motivated to raise the bar higher.

ACCOUNTABILITY.

When you surround yourself with friends that support you and have your back....you stay on track longer. You enjoy the journey. You press on.

ACCESSIBILITY.

With social media-- the lights are always on. There is always someone there to lift you up when you are feeling down or answer questions that are driving you crazy.

It's a beautiful thing to witness the transformations that occur mentally and physically every day. It makes me very proud of what we have created and I have no problem saying that The GAIN Plan and Century Club Challenge, along with the other ideas that Victor has developed, will be of interest to FitFluential community that has only just begun to change lives all over the world. And that is pretty epic indeed.

CONTENTS

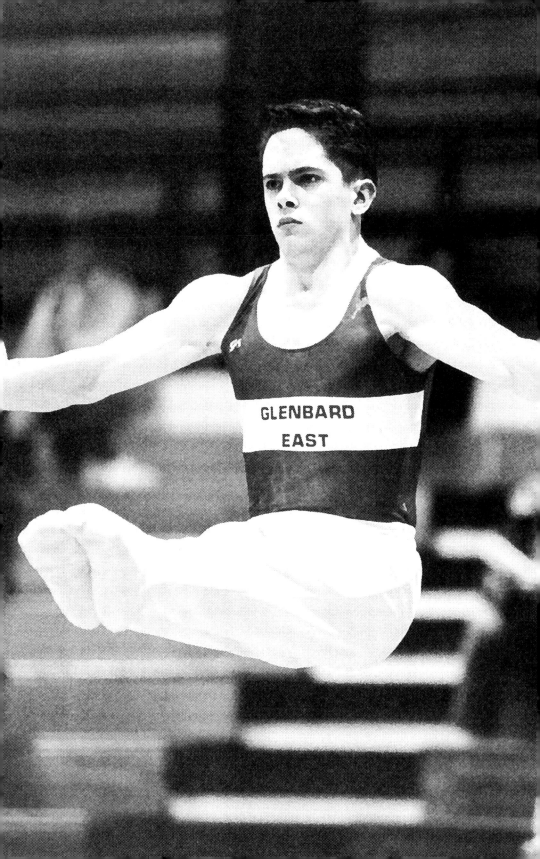

The Birth of G.A.I.N.

1. The Last Day of My Former Life

The road to success can be long and winding. Sure it sounds cliché, but goal attainment requires overcoming failure. Most of the potholes on our journey are manageable. We grow from these small challenges becoming wiser and stronger. Every once in a while we trip into a canyon of a pothole that sets us back to a place further than where we started. For me, that canyon was found on the Santa Monica boardwalk in 2005.

The journey started back in high school. In my freshman year I fell in love with the sport of gymnastics. In particular, the strength and power displayed on the still rings became my passion. You see, I was 14 years old and 110 lbs when I started gymnastics. The 9 year old girls had more muscle than me. I figured that if gymnastics could put muscle on those girls, perhaps it could put muscle on me.

With years of training in high school and college gymnastics, I achieved my goal of becoming an elite gymnast with great strength on the rings. I achieved the status of the top ranked ring specialist in the country. I would become an All-American gymnast in college. After medical school and a short hiatus from competing on the rings, I was the strongest I had ever been. I was lifting weights and training the rings 4 days a week. I built a mini ring tower in my apartment so I could train the rings any time it appealed to me. At 30 years old, I was a physical specimen.

Being a doctor and athlete caught the eye of the supplement company Muscletech and I became a sponsored athlete. I continued to train even harder splitting my attention between both weight training and gymnastics. I lost track of my physical and mental well-being. I ignored aches and soreness while becoming even more restrictive in my diet with no carbs, no fat, just protein. I was all ahead full without throttling down, ever. Pain was "weakness leaving the body" and I inflicted a lot of pain on my body in the gym.

This kind of blind ambition and reckless drive is bound to lead to a Grand Canyon sized crash. The crash would come during a magazine photo shoot. The magazine was shooting me on the rings on "Muscle Beach" Santa Monica, California. This was on old rusty metal rings over sand, very different than the ones used in gymnastics.

After a long night of orthopaedic trauma call and an equally long flight to L.A., I was ready to shoot – or so I thought. I had gotten to L.A. late that Friday evening and went to the beach at 6:00 am. The morning air was a bit chilled with a brisk wind carrying the scents of Pacific salt water to the shore. Wearing a pair of swim trunks, I headed for the rings hanging from a tall tower on the beach. I barely warmed up as I was so excited to show off in front of the camera.

As I got up on the rings, I felt great. The excitement poured strength into my arms. The photographer was still setting up his camera about 20 feet away. I jumped up to a support on the rings and looked up saying, "Watch this!" I lowered my body into a perfectly level iron-cross with my arms out to the side for about 5 seconds.

As I performed the iron cross, I effortlessly pulled myself up to a Maltese cross with my legs and body parallel to the ground like superman flying. Suddenly, I felt and heard a loud CRACK!

I instantly knew what had happened, but at that time I didn't have an appreciation for how to cope with it or even exactly why it happened. Tears welled up in my eyes. The photographer was nauseated by the sound even 20 feet away. My distal bicep tendon had torn clean off the bone. It was instantly devastating to my motivation and my dreams to be a world champion in gymnastics. I knew I would never touch the rings again. I knew I wouldn't be able to operate for at least six weeks. It would take me months to recover.

2. What Now?

I did a lot of soul searching after that event. With my gymnastics career over, I needed to start over, to develop a new passion that would restore my spirit and motivate me to return to the gym. Whatever the direction, I knew one thing; this time I would approach training differently.

Although gymnastics had held my greatest attention for years, I was always intrigued by the sport of bodybuilding. Looking for something fresh, I began to pursue bodybuilding with the same passion as I had for gymnastics. Only this time, I took time. Applying my knowledge of medicine, human physiology, and nutrition, I carefully planned my diet and exercise routines. This time I would concentrate on recovery, balanced nutrition, listening to my aches and pains, and objective evaluations of my progress.

I realized along the way why I had failed on the rings that day. I had many distractions and myths in my training that I didn't fully appreciate until preparing for bodybuilding competitions. You see, bodybuilding is truly a lifestyle. More of your success in bodybuilding occurs outside of the gym in the form of diet and recovery from training. I should've realized this more in gymnastics, but for some reason it took a tragic event to open my eyes.

The distractions are all around us in the form of multimedia, mass marketing, and false interpretation of data. I didn't realize the problems with processed, sugar laden foods. I didn't understand the mind-body-mind connection so critical to physical and mental recovery from stress and training. I self-medicated for lack of sleep with coffee. I didn't maximize my protein intake and use of dietary supplements. I thought fruits were of equal importance to vegetables. The list goes on, and my goal in this book it to prevent you from being duped.

As you can imagine, in the very conservative environment of orthopaedic surgery, involvement in bodybuilding brought on wrinkled foreheads and unsolicited comments. As I gained weight trying to build muscle all the questions started pouring in. At first it was questions about my diet. "You eat chicken breasts and broccoli every day?" "What supplements do you use?" "How often and how long do you workout?" "Can you help me get in shape?" These are all questions that I welcomed. It was these questions that helped me to refine my knowledge about my training as I never wanted to give bad advice.

Then I started doing well on the national stage. I lived the bodybuilding diet and training lifestyle every day. I didn't let it get in the way of my orthopaedic training and I was very efficient with my diet and the gym. I trained at 4:30 in the morning and 8:00 at night. I stopped at the gym on my way home from the hospital 5 days a week. As I became more successful, the troublesome questions started. "Do you like bodybuilding more than orthopaedics?" "Are you going to give up medicine if you turn pro?" "Do you use anabolic steroids?"

Whenever you become successful at something and more public with your accomplishments, the jealous naysayers pop up. Unfortunately, bodybuilding has a reputation for being on the fringe and in-conducive with being an intelligent surgeon. One of my clinical instructors was very interested in how I was getting in shape. Every day he would ask me about what I was eating and what my workouts were. He acted genuinely interested. Then on one of my evaluations he said, "I think Victor cares more about bodybuilding than orthopaedics." Here he was the one asking all the questions, getting me to talk about it, and he gave me a less than glowing evaluation for discussing bodybuilding. At that point I decided to keep most of my training to myself. However, my accomplishments spoke for themselves. My chairman only cared if you were a female football player or a marathoner and would announce their accomplishments to the department and newspapers. When I won the National Championships, there wasn't a peep. Maybe he was jealous of my accomplishment that he had nothing to do with and couldn't take any credit for?

The moral of the story is, stay true to your goals and follow your dreams no matter what others say or think about you. Those that admire your success don't love YOU, they would love to BE you. Those that stuck with you through thick and thin are the ones that LOVE you!

After 5 years of bodybuilding competition, I would eventually reach the pinnacle of my second amateur sport, winning the NPC National Championships as a welterweight bodybuilder at 36 years old. I had also become a well-respected orthopaedic surgeon with a growing practice.

3. A New Lifestyle: Recovering from Imbalance

The process of getting to the peak of my sport was exhilarating. All of the challenges and bumps in the road gave me a great sense of accomplishment. I developed the ability to change directions by refocusing my competitive spirit and life-style. And in the process, I developed a more balanced regimen of exercise, positive attitude, integrating mindfulness, Yoga and other healthy behaviors and of course, proper nutrition. I called it my *G.A.I.N. Plan*, for **G**raded Exercise, **A**ttitude, **I**ntegrated Medicine and Nutrition. Today, I continue to refocus this spirit on various physical and mental challenges. I've gone back to my gymnastics roots reinventing my exercise routines into a personal competitive sport which I call the *Century Club Challenge* that I'll share with you. And I've tried new sports and new dance styles. I'm doing all of these things with an open mind and especially open eyes; because blind ambition can run anyone into the ground.

Our bodies and mind require stimulation to grow but need equal time to recover in order to become receptive to further growth. For instance, going to the gym and lifting weights. You push hard enough to make your biceps sore. When brushing your teeth the next morning the sore biceps remind you of your hard work. If you ignore this pain and work your biceps too soon, you will increase the pain to the point where you can't even lift a toothbrush. If you don't heed the warnings you will end up like me on the rings that day.

Arnold Schwarzenegger is famous for saying that he didn't go to his father's funeral because he wouldn't let anything get in the way of his training. In the movie *Pumping Iron*, he said that if someone stole his car he wouldn't care. He was focused on the task of being Mr. Olympia.

Being in such a bubble takes a certain type of personality that not many people have. Therefore, most of us are affected by our environments. Mental stress from events like a death in the family or a stolen car leads to physical effects that can disrupt your recovery from training and decrease your ability to perform.

Studies suggest that working appropriately through life stressors improves your versatility, adaptability, resiliency, and "can-do" mindset. As long as you allow your mind and body to recover from each event without building-up "recovery debt", you can continue to be productive by plugging along. Don't hold your stress inside for too long, it will catch up to you in mental and physical fatigue.

The same happens with our minds. The stress of studying for a test helps us to learn the material better. Can you remember days of studying hard for a test? Some of those days seem like yesterday to me. However, if you throw a death in the family, a relationship breakup, and someone steals your car while you are studying for that test, your likelihood of failure increases; too much stress! As you will learn about in this book, all of that mental stress creates equally destructive stress on your body.

In order to avoid the over-load that can lead to devastation, you must approach your life and your goals in manageable pieces. Attention to this concept lead me to *G.A.I.N.*, the 4 aspects of life that need be monitored and regularly maintained to make sure that you can recognize when your body and mind are "over-stressed". **G**raded Exercise, Positive **A**ttitude, **I**ntegrated Medicine, and Balanced **N**utrition are the keys to GAINing longevity and performance. Graded exercise keeps your mind, muscles, and heart healthy. A positive attitude leads to an optimistic outlook in all aspects of life, fuels motivation and harnesses your competitive spirit with the mindset that you can still be your best. Integrated medicine and related methods of mindfulness promotes balance and self-awareness. And proper nutrition and dietary supplementation keep the mind and body ready to take on the challenges you give them. Your physical health requires a proactive agenda. As a surgeon and athlete, I've learned the hard way; prevention of medical problems is far easier than dealing with injury and disease.

4. The G.A.I.N. Plan Advantage

The *G.A.I.N. Plan* principles will teach you to adapt to change, find knowledge, break through barriers, and give you fuel for your competitive spirit. It may take some effort at first, but you will develop healthy habits that serve you for years to come. You will learn to break your tasks down into manageable pieces. You will harness your competitive spirit and your primal abilities to adapt to your world around you. You will learn ways to inspire your competitive side in the gym. You will learn to live healthier focusing on longevity in life and sport. You will learn to connect your mind to your body through monitoring your physiology. And you will learn to make your food and nutritional supplementation flexible and keep your body on target to your goals.

Use this book as a reference. Come back to it now and then to refresh your memory on the concepts and suggestions made here. Give yourself notes in the margin, sticky tags, or flags on topics that you find particularly important for you. Some of the material in this book may not pertain to you at all, whereas other parts may hit straight home. Try not to perseverate on parts that don't make sense to you. Move forward and find what speaks directly to you.

After you learn the concepts of *The G.A.I.N. Plan*, consider reading follow-up books in the *G.A.I.N.* series for your specific goals. Whether you want to lose weight, gain muscle, feel better, or live longer, The G.A.I.N. Plan will give you direction in life.

Good luck in your journey. When you realize that the road won't always be smooth, you'll be prepared for the potholes. Accept challenges that come along; change direction and G.A.I.N. from them.

The Pillars of G.A.I.N.

1. One Piece at a Time

The first time my grandmother told me, "the best way to eat an elephant is one bite at a time," my first question was, "why would anyone want to eat an elephant?" Some problems seem so large, you don't even want to start. Rebuilding my strength after my accident and focusing on another set of goals seemed insurmountable at first. But the challenge seemed less formidable when I thought about it as that elephant. The goal and the process go hand in hand. An overwhelming goal can be discouraging. Knowing there's a way to achieve the goal, one step at a time, and knowing what those steps are, makes it possible to start.

The central challenge to accomplishing any long-term goal is to have a way to stay on track. Getting stronger and living longer are big goals, and even if you get off the starting block, sustaining the effort isn't easy. Unlike a race, there is no finish line. So how do you sustain a lifelong commitment to something that has no finish line? The answer is to make a long race into a series of smaller and varied ones, each with their own challenges and goals. The importance of variety can't be understated. No matter how small the bite, if they all taste the same, eventually you loose motivation.

2. Variety

When it comes to adding variety in your life to be healthier, live longer, or perform better, it is important to take small bites with variety. Variety is truly the spice of life. You have to change things up

Chapter 1

or you will get bored. Your body needs variety so that it is constantly adapting to your environment. Your muscles grow when they see a new challenge. Variety helps to mobilize those stubborn fat stores.

By breaking your health and well-being down into four crucial pillars, *The G.A.I.N. Plan* gives you a variety of pieces to chew on in small enough bites that eventually, you can continue moving forward and enjoy it too!

3. The Four Pillars

The G.A.I.N. Plan incorporates 4 pillars of health, well-being, and performance. The pillars of *G.A.I.N.* include the concepts of :

G Graded Exercise
A Attitude
I Integrated Medicine
N Nutrition.

Each of these pillars builds the foundation for success in any lifestyle goal no matter how big or how small.

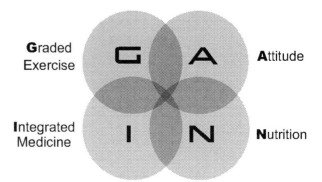

Graded Exercise   G   A   **A**ttitude

Integrated Medicine   I   N   **N**utrition

The Venn diagram on the bottom of the previous page illustrates the overlapping importance of each in personal success. In brief each one is defined as the following:

G Graded Exercise: Graded exercise refers to the two definitions of the word graded. First, exercise should be both gradual in progress as in a steady incline or "grade" with as little plateaus as possible. Second, you must "grade" your performance and monitor your progress systematically. Without a measure of progress it is very easy to lose sight of goals and feel defeated. Grading yourself objectively by body composition, strength, endurance, appearance, or physiologic markers allows you to compete with your yesterday's self; adding to competitive motivation and a sense of accomplishment.

A Attitude: Attitude is a disposition, a feeling, and a manner by which one sees the world. Feelings of defeat come from clouded and negative attitudes. The mind and thus attitude have profound effects on your physiology as the mind-body connection is very powerful. Attitude affects exercise performance and vice versa. Negative attitude can be a sign of too much training or cause you to train too little. Monitoring your attitude toward your goal attainment is critical. That being said, producing short-term successes while pacing yourself is critical to nurturing the attitude for goal attainment.

I Integrated Medicine: *The G.A.I.N. Plan* "integrates" medical knowledge and attention to health into all components of the plan. This includes the use of evidenced base medicine as well as an appreciation of alternative or nontraditional medical techniques. Learning the signs of problems and early detection of medical issues is critical to long-term well-being and attainment of performance goals. Knowing when too much is too much or too little is too little is important in avoiding illness and injury.

N **Nutrition:** Nutrition refers simply to what goes into your mouth. You are what you eat and The G.A.I.N. Plan is about you at your healthiest. You wouldn't put low octane fuel into a Ferrari, so why put it in your body? *The G.A.I.N. Plan* will teach you the keys to maximizing your longevity, performance, and recovery from exercise through proper nutrition and dietary supplementation. *The G.A.I.N. Plan* and its online applications will help you to burn fat, build muscle, and live well.

4. Pillars Must be Combined

As the Venn diagram on the previous spread illustrates, the pillars of *The G.A.I.N. Plan* cannot stand alone. Many programs try to present each of these concepts independently or as 1, 2, or 3. Without attention to all 4 pillars, a program will fail; maybe not in the short-term but definitely in the long-term. For instance, diet plans consistently fail without adequate exercise or attention to medical problems and food sensitivities. Diets also fail if you don't have a positive mental attitude that is consistent with goal achievement or you have an unaddressed addiction or emotional attachment to foods. Simply put, *The G.A.I.N. Plan* is your home for success built on a well-balanced foundation.

Everyone has unique needs when making changes in diet, exercise, or mental attitude.

The G.A.I.N. Plan for one person will have different emphasis than that for another. Everyone reading this book will have slightly different goals. You may want to be a champion bodybuilder. Perhaps you just want to see your abs again. Maybe you just want to try a new workout routine like the *Century Club Challenge*. Whatever your goal is, the foundation of achieving it must be built on the pillars of *G.A.I.N.*

My brother came to visit for Thanksgiving this past year. Having been a runner and musician, building muscle had never been a priority. However, now that he's living in a new town and is single again he wants to put on muscle. He has even considered competing in a physique contest.

For the past few months Tony had been training harder in the gym. He has tried to build muscle by lifting heavier weights. He even hired a personal trainer. He was always pretty lean with a six pack but he never trained hard shoulders and legs. Now he was, and despite his heavy training he complained that he just wasn't growing. He was very frustrated. He had hit a wall.

He started to inquire about sports supplements and testosterone boosters. At this point I had to stop him and ask more details about his training and diet. First of all, in the gym he was doing 15 to 20 repetition sets close to exhaustion but not pushing the envelope. I had to convince him to train heavier, overcome fears, and try some intensity boosting techniques. We will go over those later. The biggest problem came when I asked him about his diet.

He was eating less than 100g of protein per day with most of that in his dinner and a shake. He often skipped breakfast or had 1-2 eggs with toast and orange juice. Sometimes he would just have cereal in milk. Lunch consisted of lunch meat, fruit, and a diet drink. He would appropriately have a protein shake after his workouts and a dinner with one small chicken breast and rice or pasta. Unfortunately, this is never going to help his legs and shoulders grow! He needed much more protein, more calories, more healthy fats, and more veggies. I told him that once he got his diet in order, we will talk supplements.

As you move forward in this text, take notes, write in the margins, and take your time in assimilating the knowledge and techniques presented. Try not to get overwhelmed, do it one piece at a time. Feel free to skip around after the introduction of *The G.A.I.N. Plan* principles to find information you might need right now. For instance, you want to know about what supplements to buy, go to the "supplements" section. Use the book as a reference as you move forward.

In addition to this book, visit yourgainplan.com and track your progress, get updated information, and join the social network of "GAIN Planners". Consider not only the knowledge presented, but also try to put technology to work for you. The G.A.I.N. Plan *Monitor and phone apps will provide invaluable programing and help you to achieve a level of performance you once thought impossible.*

5. Yesterday's Self

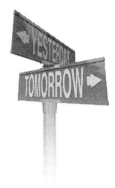

All species survive by adapting to their environment. Species that were unable to adapt to their environment, like the dinosaurs, became extinct as the world changed around them. If they weren't resilient enough to handle the stress of their environment they failed to pass on their genes. They had to fight for food, survive disease, and successfully attract the opposite sex to pass their genes down to future generations. They had to be able to adapt to their environment and become better than their "yesterday's self".

Yesterday's self is in the past, but it is your starting point. Today you need to raise the bar. You are living in the "now" and you need to challenge today's self to grow tomorrow. Tomorrow you will need to adapt again and propel yourself in a direction conducive to your goals. In essence you are constantly raising the bar and competing with yesterday's self.

When we are put into a stressful or competitive situation, we rely on a reaction in our bodies called the "Fight or Flight Response". I will discuss the specifics of this response later in the book when we talk about managing stress, but it is important to mention in order to understand our competitive nature. When we are put into a competitive situation this response revs up our minds and our bodies. We become more focused, we become more energetic, and we become more tolerant of pain. This is an innate response that both consciously and subconsciously encourages us to adapt to our environment.

You can harness the energy of the fight or flight response. When we get on a stage, it is this response that generates excitement and even a little nervousness. However, under or over-utilization of this response may cause undesired results. There is a "Goldilocks Zone" of where environmental stress revs up this response to your advantage. Remember the porridge that was too hot, too cold, or just right? Too much stress results in physical and emotional overload that disrupts your ability to perform. Too little stress results in a lack of motivation to adapt and succeed. The "just right" level of stress in the Goldilocks Zone becomes motivating and energizing. Finding this zone is the fun in your journey toward your goal. It is what you need to learn to succeed in almost all that you do.

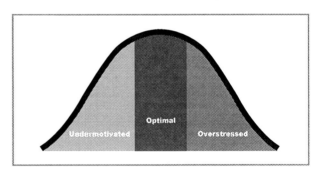

Positive Stress

By harnessing the energy of "positive stress", you can stay competitive and productive to triumph over yesterday's self. I refer to competitive drive as positive stress. It pushes you to adapt and grow in response to your environment. Adapting to your environment means that you are becoming a better person in body and mind than you were yesterday. This may also include overcoming "negative stress". Let's face it, bad things happen. It is inevitable that your environment is going to change; this will happen by choice or by chance. However, chance favors the prepared mind. By following *The G.A.I.N. Plan* you will be prepared to handle physical and mental change and recognize when adaptive change is needed.

When you are training toward a goal, whether it is building muscle, maintaining your health, or burning fat, you need to make daily changes to continue improving upon yesterday's self. Today you are a day older than yesterday. Today you may have aches and pains that you didn't have yesterday because of yesterday's workout. Today you may have gotten less sleep than yesterday. Today you might be feeling a cold coming on. Today you might have a project due at work. If you don't adapt your yesterday's self to today, your physical and mental growth will stagnate or regress tomorrow. You need to appreciate that today's self is different than yesterday's self and today presents a chance to grow and adapt in a positive way. *The G.A.I.N. Plan* will provide you with tools to recognize what changes are needed and how to make those changes day to day and week to week.

This doesn't always mean that you need to work harder than yesterday. It is very easy to get into the misguided mentality that you just need to work harder to make improvements upon your body and mind. Don't get me wrong, it does take work, but it doesn't necessarily need to be harder. It needs to be more guided and efficient. For instance, athletes often get into the trouble of under or over training when they are preparing for a competition. This only occurs when the athlete is unable to comprehend the difference between too little and too much effort. If you ask a national champion how they felt in the weeks leading up their win, they will often tell you that they just found their groove or were "in the zone". I certainly felt this way going into the NCAA Championships and the NPC National Championships. I was in a place where I was doing everything just right. I was training hard, but getting proper rest. I was eating what my body needed to recover from workouts. I was controlling my mental stress through visualization and relaxation techniques. Looking back, everything was done just right.

The competitive spirit is ingrained in all of us and all that is around us. Some of us thrive on competing with others. For those who don't like to compete with others, think about competing with your yesterday's self. To have personal growth you need to strive to be better than yesterday's self every day. You don't need to make drastic changes each day, just little ones. Push a little more weight in the gym. Eat a few more veggies. Meditate for 5 minutes. Smile more. It doesn't take much to make improvements.

I like to bring out my competitive spirit by imagining that I am on a stage performing or preparing to go on stage with whatever I'm doing. If I am doing dips, I think about the next time someone might challenge me to a dipping contest. Sometimes I'll video myself with the intention of posting it on Instagram. I know that thousands of people could potentially see that video. I won't be a slouch on that video. I want to win. We all want to win.

P.A.C.E.
*P*erformance *A*s a *C*ompetitive *E*vent

The G.A.I.N. Plan will put forth knowledge and techniques that will promote health while taking your performance to the next level. Performance can be defined in 3 ways:

a. Presentation

b. Effectiveness

c. Technique

The concept of "presentation" may or may not be remote to you. The first thing that usually comes to mind is dancers or the symphony. However, we would like to suggest that "presentation" can refer to any activity that puts you on a stage, whether that is the dance hall, in front of others in the gym, or social networking. Instagram, Twitter, and Facebook generate a world stage for you to perform.

Second, performance refers to work "effectiveness". When a job is done, it needs to be assessed for completeness and quality of the work. The same premise holds true for goals related to your health and physique; if you fail to progress toward your goals you get an F, if you reach the pinnacle of success in your discipline you get an A+.

Third, as"technique" performance refers to how well someone or something succeeds at their displaying their discipline. This has everything to do with perseverance, goal achievement, and following the rules.

The concept of P.A.C.E. comes from a combination of performing, maximizing performance, and adding competitive spirit to your goals in an effective way. When we are competing, especially in front of others, we are motivated to perform at our best. Records are broken when you compete with others. The Olympics brings out numerous American and World Records because athletes peak for the greatest stage on earth and harness the excitement to their advantage. Those who win at these contests know how to pace their training to peak at the right time.

I recommend that you utilize the "performance" aspect of achieving your goals. By performing for others you put your best foot forward. By creating your own audience you can generate the motivational energy that professional athletes get on stage. You don't necessarily have to compete against others, as long as you are competing with yesterday's self. In setting short-term daily goals you need to define who you were yesterday and what constitutes a better self today. By sharing your goals with those around you, you will create your own audience and cheering section. That audience will let you know if you are a winner!

Present challenges to other *G.A.I.N.* challengers and your yesterday's self by utilizing the social tools and record keeping applications with yourgainplan.com.

6. Unleashing the Competitor Within

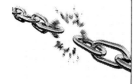

Everybody has a competitive side. Even if you don't feel like a competitive person you can harness your competitive spirit. Consider these ways to bring out your competitive side:

1. Enter a Contest

Whatever your goal might be, there's probably a contest for it. It may be a "biggest loser challenge", a bodybuilding show, or a weightlifting competition. By entering a contest, you feel the excitement of the coming event; you may even feel the pressure to win. You may just be entering a 5k run to compete with yourself by reaching a new personal best. The energy of the other runners around you will push you to new levels.

See Mindfulness Page 80

During contest prep your desire to succeed brings on the "fight or flight" stress response. Harnessing the energy of this response will boost your daily workouts and motivate you to stay on target. Whenever I prepared for a bodybuilding show, gymnastics meet, or dance performance the little bit of stress to perform well in front of others kept me focused and motivated. As you move forward in your contest prep use visualization techniques and mindfulness. See yourself on stage during each workout to maintain the excitability to perform your best.

2. Make a Contest

In the event that you can't find a contest, make a contest for yourself. All you need is a set of rules, a scoring system, and a prize. The contest could be losing 2 pounds by the end of the week. The rules might be that you aren't going to have sugars or deserts, you'll have to do 30 minutes of cardio each morning on an empty stomach, and you'll have to weigh in each morning. Follow the rules and you win a cheat meal on Sunday.

Present a challenge or a bet to a friend, colleague, or social media BFF. If you have a friend who has a similar goal bet them that you'll do it first. Hopefully they will accept your challenge and let the games begin. If your challenge is too unreasonable for you or your friend to win then you need to reassess your goals. When you challenge a friend, you may discover for the first time that your goals are unreasonable. This will be eye-opening and allow you to reset the bar for success.

3. Watch a Contest

I still get a competitive feeling when I watch gymnasts on the rings. When I see a guy doing strength moves that I used to perform, I get sweaty palms because I want to get out there and show them what I can (or could) do. Whenever I have entered a new sport or endeavor, I have observed the best in action first. Before I ever competed in bodybuilding I went to a national level show to see if it was something I could be competitive in. I met my wife at one of these shows, so there are other benefits to watching. I also shadowed an orthopaedic surgeon before going into orthopaedics. I went to dance performances and watched the best perform until I had a good visual in my mind about the style and rhythm. Watching others succeed at similar goals gives you confidence and forms a mental image of your own personal success.

7. The Century Club Challenge

If you are looking for a new physical and mental challenge, I present to you my *Century Club Challenge* (CCC). The CCC is a grueling workout that should be looked at as a strength and endurance contest with your body and mind. Of course, you could also compete with others, but this is about your personal growth, development, and sense of accomplishment.

The CCC is meant to:
1. Teach you to apply the principles of *G.A.I.N.* to a new goal.
2. Create short and long-term performance goals.
3. Build a solid foundation of strength, balance, and flexibility.
4. Generate some competitive spirit.

The CCC is not meant to be a daily or even weekly workout. In essence, this is a workout that would lead to severe over-training in most people. It is a challenge that you prepare for just as you would for a 5K, 10k, or Marathon. You need to use the *G.A.I.N. Plan* principles to build attainable goals, achieve adequate recovery, and monitor progress.

It tests your endurance, strength, and mental fortitude. It teaches you how important it is to recover from your training and avoid injury. The challenge is made such that your preparation and completion of the exercises improves your core strength, balance, bone density, flexibility, cardiovascular health, and mental toughness when done in conjunction with *The G.A.I.N. Plan's* principles.

The CCC consists of 100 repetitions of each of 10 fundamental exercises (1000 reps) performed in a variety of sequences and forms. You "join the club" by completing the exercises in under 1 hour. The fundamental exercises are meant to be done with

The Century Club Challenge Exercises

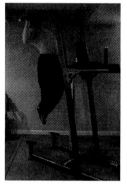

1. Chin ups/Pull Ups

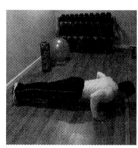

2. Push Ups

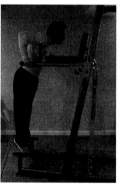

3. Parallel Bar Dips

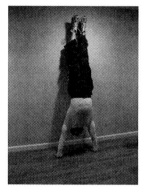

4a. Handstand Push Ups

Scan this QR code for detailed descriptions of the Century Club Challenge *exercises at* yourgainplan.com

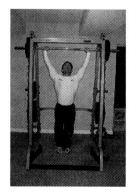

4b. Military Press

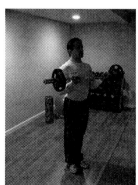

5. Barbell Curls

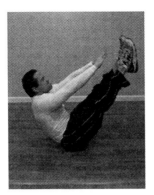

6. V-Ups

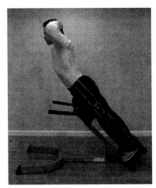

7. Back Extensions

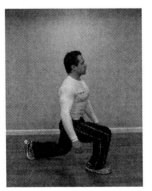

8. Alternating
Lunge Jumps

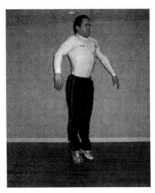

9. Squat Jumps

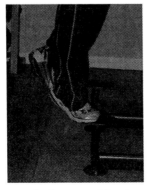

10. Single Leg Calf Raises

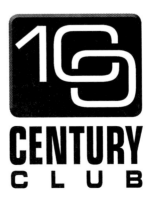

CENTURY
C L U B

strict form avoiding risk for injury and focusing on balance and conditioning of your core muscles. The CCC can be done at many levels with handicapping as needed to get through the challenge.

Please note: This is like training for a marathon. The CCC is a strength and endurance challenge that takes months, if not years, of training to accomplish. Move forward with proper progressions.

Club Levels of Century Challengers

• If you need assistance to get through the workout at any repetition level (i.e. assisted chins, kneeling pushups, etc.) you are a CCC Bronze.

• If you are able to perform all of the core exercises without assistance but not up to the full 100 reps you are a CCC Silver ¼, ½, or ¾ (denoted $Silver_{25}$, $Silver_{50}$, or $Silver_{75}$).

• If you are able to complete the full 100 repetitions of all 10 exercises you are CCC Gold.

• If you are a Gold level CC Challenger and you can add weight (i.e. weighted vest) or perform more difficult variations on the core exercises (i.e. Burpee Chin Ups) you become a CCC Platinum.

Later in the book we will go over the CCC in more detail. You can also read *The Century Club Challenge* which has more detailed workouts and tips to reach new levels of performance.

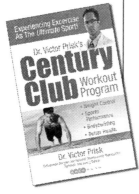

Along with the guiding principles of *The G.A.I.N. Plan*, *The Century Club Challenge* has evolved over the past 10 years to help amateur and professional athletes as well as performing artists get more satisfaction from exercise based on the premise that exercise can be practiced more safely, productively and enjoyably when it is seen as a game and a performance with an audience. Over the past decade, I have been refining these elements with various groups of athletes, performers, members of health clubs and fitness enthusiasts, who have found that its principles, even in the most primitive forms, have enhanced their lives and performance in their chosen professions or other endeavors. Their experience and prompting has encouraged a fuller look at P.A.C.E.

Communities like Crossfit have embraced a similar concept by making workouts a competition. However, the complexity and risk associated with Crossfit has given many people, such as myself, great concerns. An over emphasis on the brutality of their challenges and the lack of rigorous attention to core and form have brought a lot of negative attention to the sport of Crossfit with injury rates as great as 50% of participants in my experience. I believe Crossfitters can get back on track with strict attention to the pillars of *G.A.I.N.*

Using the structure of games to enhance the pleasure of an activity is not a new idea, but one that has been employed in education of all forms and recently, in many fields through the use of gaming technology. In the case of fitness, we see exercise as a competitive sport with a growing missionary national base.

A sport, in this sense, is an activity where participants adhere to a standard set of guiding principles, rules, scoring and handicapping elements such as classes and levels of play that allow participants of various skill levels to compete. In addition, the competitive gaming element is enhanced through recognition for achievement, club and regional tournaments and regulatory principles that ensure the safety and integrity of the sport.

The Century Club Challenge epitomizes the basic structure of P.A.C.E. connecting Century Challengers via personal and online tracking.

The Basic Structure of the Contest Consists of:

- 2 or More Competing Parties that Ensure Accurate Tracking

    – This can be you vs. others or you vs. yesterday's self

- 10 Simple to Execute Exercises with Variations that Allow Handicapping and Creativity

- A Time Constraint

- Levels of Intensity for Reps, Speed, Rest, or Number of Excrcises

- Biometric Measures Like Heart Rate

- Ratings for Each Performance Level by Club (Bronze, Silver, Gold)/community/region

Rules and Integrity

"A man has integrity if his interest in the good of the service is at all times greater than his personal pride, and when he holds himself to the same line of duty when unobserved as he would follow if his superiors were present."

– Brigadier General S.L.A. Marshall

When it comes to competition, there are almost always rules. Rules make competition fair and help identify cheaters. There are always ways to break the rules and cheat. However, those who break the rules have to live with the guilt and negative consequences if they get caught.

You may be having a competition with your yesterday's self to lose weight. You set out with rules like, I'm going to exercise more and I'm going to eat less carbohydrates. Then one day you have a cheat meal of ice-cream and cookies. You feel guilty, you feel you need to skip a meal, you feel the need to take a diet pill, and you may just want to throw up.

One way to help you maintain integrity is to think that someone is always watching you. I'm not suggesting that you become psychotic; I'm saying that you maintain integrity by acting in a way that you would as if someone else was watching. This is just like acting as though you are always performing on a stage. If you are at home alone eating a whole pumpkin pie, would you do the same if your wife was watching? Pumpkin season always gets me in trouble. If you are at the gym and your trainer wasn't watching would you stop the treadmill 10 minutes early?

Whatever it takes for you to maintain integrity and follow the rules, just do it. When you follow the rules and win in a competition you feel a greater sense of accomplishment. If you run a race and take a short cut, the win won't feel as good. You will always know that you cheated. In fact, others may have seen you cheat, but they probably won't say anything directly to you. You'll just be propagating a lie that destroys your reputation.

Play fair, play with integrity, but play to win!

Healthy Myths

The injury I sustained on Muscle Beach was due to misguidance. You would think that as a physician, experienced gymnast, and well published author on fitness that I would be immune to such a destructive injury.

In reality, I had been misguided my whole life. There were a number of myths that distracted me from maximizing my recovery and performance. These myths had been perpetuated by societal norms, bad science, and political agendas.

Why do you need to learn the principles of *The G.A.I.N. Plan*? It is likely that you have also been misguided on healthy living. As a child, did you think that a hamburger, fries, and a Coke constituted a healthy dinner? Even worse, that Frosted Flakes and OJ were the essential components of "this complete breakfast"? Were you told that all you have to do was work hard and I would succeed? Was there any talk of efficiency and networking? Needless to say, much of this influence puts us a little behind in developing skills for health, longevity, and goal attainment.

Myth #1: Pain Is Weakness Leaving The Body.

I believed that every time I went to the gym I had to give 110% effort. I thought that I had to be sore every day. I approached my training with the need to lift more every time went to the gym. I didn't realize the importance of Graded Exercise. I didn't realize that I needed to be objective in my progress and make gradual and deliberate progressions.

Constant physical stress with inadequate rest results in recovery debt. Your muscles and tendons experience damage with intense exercise. A little damage is expected and tolerable if the tissues are given time to heal. For instance the delayed onset muscle soreness you experience after a heavy workout is a sign of tissue damage. With proper recovery through rest, nutrition, and stretching your tissues heal, adapt, and become stronger. If you ignore the pain and blindly push forward, recovery debt accumulates and injuries occur. You must plan your recovery and rest just as much as you should carefully plan your workout schedule.

Myth #2: Fat-free Foods Are Good For Me.

Dr. Ancel Keys started his "Seven Countries" study in the 1950's and later concluded that saturated fat and cholesterol in the diet led to heart disease and early death. The objective was to encourage healthier eating to improve hearth health and lose body fat.

In the 1980's this data, which was inherently flawed statistically and in research methodology, led to policy changes by the U.S. Department of Agriculture. It was recommended that saturated fat intake be drastically reduced.

To replace the palatability imparted by fat, manufacturers increased the sugar content of foods. The use of widely available and cheap high fructose corn syrup became the norm in food manufacturing. Hydrogenated vegetable oils, "trans-fats", were used to replace the saturated animal fats.

Unfortunately, these policies didn't improve the health of Americans. In fact, the rates of obesity, diabetes, heart disease, and other lifestyle diseases continued to rise. We are just now beginning to realize the mistakes made in the 80's. As we will discuss further, we have come to realize the toxic and addictive nature of sugar. Public policy has changed to eliminate trans-fats from food manufacturing.

Myth #3: I Should Eat 3 Meals Per Day: Breakfast, Lunch, and Dinner.

We are all raised on the idea that 3 meals per day is the norm. This is a societal norm. Most employers give a lunch break. This is just how it was always done. However, recent research suggests that we may be better off consuming more frequent meals to improve our muscle's recovery from exercise.

When I was a resident, I ate meals only when I could. Often this was a breakfast and a dinner and I was lucky if I was able to get in a lunch. With the stress and lack of sleep, my muscle was starving for a growth stimulus that rarely came.

Myth #4: All Proteins Are Created Equal.

Although the RDA recommends only 0.8g/kg body weight of protein per day, organizations like the American College of Sports Medicine and The International Society for Sports Nutrition have made it fairly clear that resistance trained athletes need closer to 2.0g/kg body weight per day.

*Get the
G.A.I.N. Plan
App to
maximize
your
Leucine*

However, a recent study showed that most Americans eat there protein skewed more towards the evening meal. In other words, most people eat 10g of protein with breakfast, 15g of protein with lunch and 65g of protein with dinner. The researchers decided to see what happened to muscle growth if the protein was more evenly distributed across meals (30g x 3 meals). What they found was that the evenly distributed protein led to more muscle growth.

Clearly, there was a threshold for muscle growth that wasn't being reached with the breakfast and lunch protein content in the skewed diets. As it turns out there is a stimulus that wasn't being reached. Furthermore, other researchers have shown that proteins like whey isolates have a greater muscle growth response than equal amounts of soy protein or wheat protein.

It turns out that all proteins aren't created equal. However, the RDA doesn't make this distinction. Proteins are made of amino acids found in various ratios that make the proteins distinct. It just so happens that whey protein isolates are very high in the branched-chain amino acid, L-leucine. Leucine is an amino acid found in larger quantities in muscle proteins and has distinct actions on muscle protein synthesis.

In fact, leucine acts as a molecular key to turn on the machinery that builds muscle proteins from leucine and other amino acids. Studies suggest that consuming 0.04mg/kg body weight per meal will maximize your muscle protein synthesis. So, why not follow the leucine content of your food if you want to maximize your lean muscle. Food for thought. We will go over this in the Nutrition section in more detail.

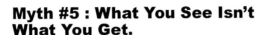

Myth #5 : What You See Isn't What You Get.

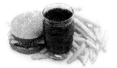

How many times have you seen a commercial where a fast food restaurant presents you with this "complete" meal: a cheeseburger, fries, and a Coke? Those of us with some nutritional savvy and fitness acumen can't be fooled by this sort of marketing. To my dismay kids and some adults just don't realize this.

It literally makes me viscerally sick to think of such a meal as a lunch or dinner. It makes me even sicker how long I fell for this marketing and had this for lunch. Up until my injury and road to bodybuilding success I would regularly grab a lunch at a fast food joint. Now when I see that food I am thoroughly disgusted. *The G.A.I.N. Plan* was created to bring this to the attention of more people. Food marketing gives us a false sense of what is healthy and nutritious, thus we need to educate ourselves and others to avoid being taken advantage of by big business.

For the first time in history, lifestyle diseases like diabetes, heart disease, strokes, and some cancers kill more people than communicable diseases. Most of us don't even realize that our life-styles are creating this problem. Patients always say to me that they are overweight and out of shape because of their genetics. Patients will say to me, "I eat healthy, I just have a slow metabolism". Meanwhile they're holding a 20 oz regular soft drink and can't even tell me what they had for breakfast, lunch, and dinner the day before.

I don't always blame the patient for this attitude. This is because many just don't know any better, and the world around them doesn't make it any easier. Unfortunately, media exposure in the form of advertisements, TV commercials, and even the evening news can be incredibly confusing and misleading.

I made *The G.A.I.N. Plan* to guide you away from all the distractions in everyday life that drag you away from your goals. *The G.A.I.N. Plan* provides a scientific basis for doing things that will help you achieve your goals. It elaborates on how exercise done in a graded fashion will add years to your life and life to your years. I will show you how a 5-M.A.D. diet and nutritional supplementation can improve your energy, longevity, and strength. I will describe ways that you can work with your doctors or therapists to practice preventative medicine and recognize your genetic risks. Perhaps most importantly, *The G.A.I.N. Plan* will help you to have an attitude which propels you toward your goals and health without hesitation or distraction.

We are living in an age of distraction where the world around us wants to divert our attention from our personal development. Let's start working on your *G.A.I.N. Plan* right now. To start, grab a sheet of paper. Start by writing down your daily distractions. Are you using Facebook to email and communicate with others, or are you trying to escape the real world? Perhaps you're just looking to see if your life is better than someone else's? Is your cell phone a distraction? Do you have a friend that makes you go to the bars too often? Does someone else in your house buy a lot of junk food? Do you turn on the TV as soon as you walk in the door?

My Daily Distractions:

_____

_____

_____

_____

_____

_____

_____

_____

_____

Now that you have written down your distractions, try and estimate how much time you give attention to each distraction in a given day. Once you have the total time calculated, make another list. This list is a list of things you think you could accomplish if you had all that time added on to your day. Don't forget to add some time for reading _The G.A.I.N. Plan_, as this is definitely going to be a life changing experience.

Myth #6 : Genes Don't Lie.

There are always articles and newscasts that try to bring attention to your genes as the source of your fat, your appetite, and your muscle mass. The media spin always plays the blame game on your genes. "Defective gene for Leptin causes obesity" "The hunger hormone gene Ghelin causes you to become fat". The headlines and teasers can be like, "Did you know your genes can make you fat? More at 5." In essence they turn new scientific discoveries into marketing tools to bring more people to the television or to buy their newspaper.

Furthermore they twist the information to make you feel better. If you are overweight and someone tells you that it's not your fault it's your parent's fault (your genes) it takes the responsibility for your weight off your shoulders. In reality, your environment and your daily decision making lead to your excessive weight. Ignore the news twist on science and have intellectual discussions with your physician or analyze the data yourself.

We are always hearing about how so many diseases and disorders have a genetic basis. In fact, we see it on the news almost every day. For instance, a study comes out that says people are genetically inclined to be obese, or to smoke, drink, or have diabetes. When people hear that it must be their genetics causing their problem, they assume it is out of their control. Media sources know that people like to hear that their problems are genetic. We feel better hearing these stories as they just wash our hands of personal responsibility for our health problems. We say, "See it's my parents' fault that I'm overweight."

Clearly this is flawed reasoning in many ways. First, these studies are intended to recognize genetics as a risk factor so that if your parents had a disease, you'll work harder on disease prevention. In reality, only 1/3rd of aging is really related to our genes. Our environment has a much greater impact unless you have a rare life-threatening genetic disorder. Second, the studies presented by the newspaper and the evening news are being interpreted by one reporter or news agency and may be loaded with agendas or advertising dollars.

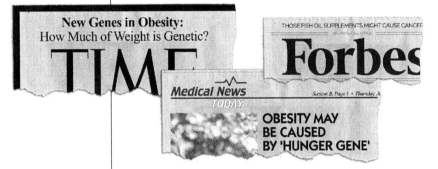

Even a study with no scientific merit can make it in the news if the headline is sensational enough to attract viewers. "Chocolate cures skin cancer!" "Coffee causes prostate cancer!" "Your multivitamin might kill you!" If you saw a teaser for the 5 O'clock news with one of those stories, wouldn't you want to watch?

The numbers don't lie when it comes to environmental stress and our greatest health problems. Environmental factors have been identified as up to 90% of the cause of the three of the most dominant chronic health conditions afflicting Americans: diabetes type II, coronary heart disease, and most site-specific cancers. There is a dramatic shift in the preponderance of such conditions as scientists think these were very rare in the Paleolithic man.

There is unequivocal evidence in the literature supporting the notion that all environmental factors combined, including physical inactivity, account for the majority of chronic health conditions. A Scandinavian twin study showed that greater than 68% of site-specific cancers had an environmental origin. The Harvard Center for Cancer Prevention estimated that, of the total number of cancer deaths, 30% were due to tobacco, 30% to adult diet and obesity, 5% to occupational factors, and 2% to environmental pollution.

In another study of 84,000 female nurses, 91% of the cases of Type 2 diabetes and 82% of the coronary artery disease cases could be attributed to bad habits and so-called "high risk behavior". The high risk behaviors included in the study were being overweight, eating a diet low in fiber and high in unhealthy trans-fat, sugar exposure, living a sedentary lifestyle, and smoking. Simply put, the majority of deaths from chronic health conditions in the United States are of environmental origin. That is, an origin that *you can control*!

Physical inactivity or what I call "activity deficiency" is the third leading cause of death in the United States. Sedentary living further contributes to the second leading cause of death, obesity. This accounts for at least 1 in 10 deaths. In fact, studies show that up to 50% of all cases of Type 2 diabetes, coronary heart disease, and many cancers can be prevented by 30 min of moderate-intensity exercise each day.

Treating these diseases — and the futile attempts to "cure" them — costs a fortune, more than 1/7th of our gross domestic product (GDP)! That is 1/7th of all the goods and services produced by the U.S. at any given time! The crazy thing is that these are diseases that can be prevented by doing things that cost no extra money. You prevent them by making healthy changes in your lifestyle.

See Brown Adipose Tissue Page 257

If you have a sedentary job, you will have less Non-Exercise Activity Thermogenesis (NEAT). NEAT is the generation of body heat throughout the day which is a large portion of your calorie burn. Special fat cells called brown fat can generate a lot of this heat by burning your fat stores. It is important to realize that exercise is not the only way to burn calories. When we sit more, we can turn the brown fat on by lowering the room temperature (65 degrees F), eating protein rich low sugar foods, and using supplements like pepper extracts. You can control your environment and overcome almost any genetic predisposition.

Are there lurking negative effects of sitting idle during the work day? Statistics say yes! Bus drivers and those sitting at telephones have nearly twice the rate of cardiovascular disease as those with standing and walking jobs. Research shows that there's a progressive inverse relationship between risk for death from all causes and non-exercise activity in women. This means the more active you are, regardless of whether you take time to exercise, the longer you will live. There is clearly an impact of inactivity on human health on the level with smoking or high cholesterol. We should treat "Activity Deficiency" with the same fervor as vitamin D deficiency, smoking risks, and dyslipidemia.

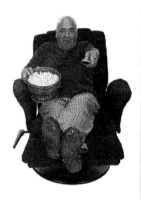

Epigenetics

How is a sedentary lifestyle a potent environmental trigger for the development of chronic health conditions? Environmental factors are thought to exert their influence by altering the expression genes protecting you from pathologic states. This effect is discussed explained by "epigenetics". Physical inactivity is an environmental factor that effects the expressions of genes needed for healthy metabolism. Modern humans are still genetically adapted to a pre-agricultural hunter-gatherer life-style, because our overall genetic makeup has changed little during the past 10,000 years. Hunter-gatherer societies likely had to undertake moderate physical activity for more than 30 min each day to provide basic necessities, such as food, water, shelter, materials for warmth, and so forth, to survive.

One might presume any gene that didn't support an active lifestyle would have resulted in natural selection of that gene to die off. On the other hand, a gene that would support moderate physical activity by allowing a greater capacity to fuel physical work would have been more likely to survive, and its gene pool would be transferred to future generations. Thus it is likely that many metabolic features of modern humans evolved as an adaptation to a physically active lifestyle, coupled with a diet high in protein and low in fat, interspersed with frequent periods of famine.

The concept of cycles of feast and famine engendered Neel's "thrifty gene" hypothesis. According to this hypothesis, those individuals with "thrifty" metabolic adaptations would convert more of their calories into stored fat during periods of feasting. As a consequence, those with the thrifty genes would be less likely to be eliminated during periods of famine.

Being able to adapt to famine is obviously beneficial to survival. Your body's metabolism or energy expenditure fluxes during feast or famine. A reduction in energy intake below necessity results in a series of physiological, biochemical, and behavioral responses to adapt and survive. One of these adaptations is "atrophy" of muscle where muscle protein is degraded as a source for glucose production by the liver. Starvation is also associated with a spontaneous decrease in daily physical activity from mental and physical fatigue. This results in even further breakdown of muscle, because there isn't a stimulus to keep the muscle. (You don't use it you lose it). Muscle is a very metabolically active tissue that consumes a lot of energy. By using it for fuel during starvation, you not only have a fuel source but you stop using up the fuel.

Physical inactivity is an abnormal event for a genome programmed to expect physical activity, thus explaining, in part, the genesis of how physical inactivity leads to metabolic dysfunctions and eventual metabolic disorders such as atherosclerosis, hypertension, obesity, Type 2 diabetes, etc. It can be easily guessed that the caloric expenditure of daily physical activity is much less today than in the hunter-gatherer society. The 30 min of moderate exercise daily in present guidelines results in expenditure of only 44% of the calories of two 20th century hunter-gatherer societies and is far below the amount of activity that our genes are programmed to expect. Consequently a mismatch between our ancient genes and our daily lives becomes a disadvantage to the sedentary individual with easy access to food. Sedentary individuals store fat in anticipation of a famine that does not come because food is available on demand. Some of those who develop obesity and Type 2 diabetes likely have the genes necessary for survival as a caveman. They store fat well and are able to keep blood sugar levels high (diabetes) even in times of relative famine (elevated fasting glucose levels).

Aging in a sedentary lifestyle leads to loss of muscle and weakness that comes with increased chance of falling and thus having a hip, spine, or wrist fracture. From the second to the eighth decade of life muscle mass can decrease by more than 25% leading to difficulties with walking, showering, and caring for personal needs. That loss of lean body mass also results in a decrease in basal metabolic rate which lowers need for food or increases storage of excess food as fat.

Chronic disease presents a heavy burden to society, in terms of both medical costs and human suffering. The good news is that readily available exercise is the most effective weapon in our arsenal in the war on chronic disease. The bad news is that exercise and its benefits are the least used weapons in our arsenal. I believe that medical community under prescribes exercise. It's not that doctors don't tell patients that they need to exercise, but they don't actually prescribe a plan for exercise. Doctors like myself need to change the way we suggest exercise and get more specific. Exercise attacks the roots of chronic disease deeply seated in activity deficiency. Exercise maintains muscle and muscle keeps us healthy.

Myth #7: The OJ Conundrum

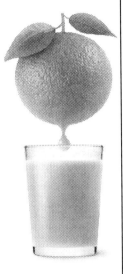

It always amazes me how Orange Juice (OJ) manufactures try to sell the "natural goodness" of OJ. The photos often show the juice coming straight from the sun or right off the tree itself. They include green leaves to make it appear more diversified in its nutritional value. Don't be fooled, OJ is sugar water that can lead you down the road of metabolic dysfunction!

Let's take media distractions a step further. Commercials from our childhood make an indelible impression on our minds that marketers take advantage of on a regular basis. The root of this evil comes in the form of breakfast cereal commercials. Let's be clear from the start, breakfast cereal with milk doesn't make a complete breakfast even if you add a slice of toast and a glass of orange juice. "Part of this complete breakfast", I think not.

A big problem arises from these commercials in the form of a tall glass of orange juice. Orange juice commercials make their juice look like pure energy from the Florida sun ready to fuel your body. But seriously, how much nutrition is in an 8 oz glass of OJ? Water, sugar, vitamin C, folate, thiamin, antioxidants, and some added nutrients from processed brands (such as calcium and vitamin D). Even though the antioxidant and vitamin content may be of value, if I added these nutrients to a can of regular Coke would you still consider this a nutritious part of this "balanced" breakfast? Sugar and water are the main ingredients supplied by nature. If you read a food label that had the first ingredient water and the second ingredient sugar, would you find it nutritious? If you would, you need to keep reading.

To understand the effect that sugars have on our metabolism, we will have to go over a little of the physiology. When you drink a glass of OJ, or sugar water for that matter, there is a rather rapid rise in blood sugar levels in your blood because the sugar (glucose) from the OJ is rapidly absorbed. When sugar levels are high, it is important that your body clear it from the blood fairly rapidly as the sugar can cause damage to tissues (seen as complications of diabetes: kidney disease, vascular disease, neuropathy, etc). Insulin is the hormone responsible for getting the sugar out of the blood and putting it into tissues like the liver, fat, or muscle. As a result of drinking rapidly absorbed sugar water, insulin is released equally as rapidly to help clear it from the blood.

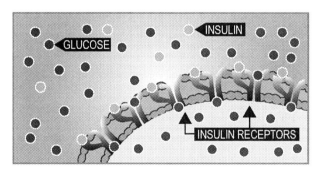

After a night's sleep your sugar stores in the liver (glycogen stores) are depleted from the fasting. Your first meal replenishes some of the glycogen stores used up during the overnight fast. Once those stores are replete, the rest that isn't expended as energy in the form of activity is converted into and stored as fat.

Since OJ causes a rapid rise in insulin (the "insulin spike") it also causes a rapid decrease in blood sugar levels. When this sugar is cleared rapidly we feel the "crash". That is a rather rapid decrease in energy level and an increase in hunger. We feel tired, sluggish, jittery, and begin to crave sweets. By this time you have driven to work and started your day. You get to work and now you're hungry, but you didn't bring a snack.

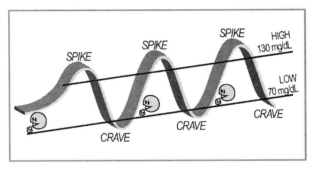

However, your cubicle mate and the vending machine down the hall have a fine selection of sugary snacks. So you eat some of this sweet delight. Now you spike your insulin again and the cycle of cravings is perpetuated. You get to lunch with another valley in your blood sugar and you eat more than you should because you're even hungrier! More spikes occur throughout your day. These high blood levels of insulin over years with lack of physical activity can lead to a decrease in your body's sensitivity to insulin. It's like becoming tolerant of a drug. You need more sugar and insulin to get an effect. You will see in further sections that sugar really can be a toxic drug.

Your body adapts to its environment. When something is thrown at it too much, it decreases its sensitivity to it. Your hands build up callouses when you work hard. Or even worse, a drug addict needs more and more pain medicine when they abuse it because they build up a tolerance. The intolerance to insulin, or decreased "insulin sensitivity", and eventual burnout of the pancreas which makes insulin is the basis for type II diabetes. This form of diabetes is on the rise in our country and is a major contributor to death and disability in the U.S.

When you go to the grocery store and you see "juice" products they don't sound so healthy anymore, do they? But many people don't realize this and the marketing world takes advantage of us. We struggle with our diets because marketers and manufacturers take advantage of our healthy connotations by over utilizing things like the word "juice". We struggle with food choices and we fail at our diets, when it really isn't our fault. We are misled down a path of "healthy" and "natural" and "wholesome" foods that ruin our goals to be lean.

OJ and the "Natural Lie"

Most people understand that we have way too many additives in our foods and many parents are worried that these processed foods can be bad for a developing child. There is a big push these days for "natural" foods. If you go to the the natural foods market, you will find it hard to find a cereal box with the ingredients "high fructose corn syrup" (HFCS). Syrup is a sweet treat that comes from maple trees and is just a sugary condiment for pancakes. Not healthy enough for my child, right? Besides, there's been enough bad press about HFCS that it has a bad connotation in itself as a processed "chemical" in foods.

In fact, studies have implicated fructose (a sugar found in many fruits) in many health problems including cancer. Fructose is metabolized differently in the liver leading to easier conversion to fat and a delay in satiety causing over-eating. To distract you from this bad press, marketing folks and natural food makers have decided to call their sugar "evaporated cane juice". Now you have a cereal that is made out of a juice that is "naturally" evaporated from something grown "cane".

Evaporated cane juice is a loosely defined term which can include combinations of sugars including glucose and fructose. Although it is less processed than bleached white sugar, the nutritional benefits are minimal. Evaporated cane juice contains trace minerals and vitamins but has the same amount of calories as table sugar. The U.S. Food and Drug Administration defines evaporated cane juice as any sweetener derived from sugar cane syrup. Although evaporated cane juice does carry miniscule amounts of nutrients, it's important to note that both are still high in the sugar sucrose (combo of glucose and fructose= table sugar), which when consumed excessively is stored in the body as fat.

If a manufacturer put "sugar" as the second ingredient to the complex carbohydrate (corn, rice, or wheat), no parent would think that would be healthy for their child or themselves. But many think, "Juice is better for my child, I know that because OJ is so healthy! ". You will no longer be distracted by such gibberish! Just look at how a Post Cereals changed the name of Sugar Crisp to Golden Crisp. Sugar obviously has unhealthy connotations and the change in name helped boost sales. The focus of Post's advertising shifted from targeting just children to including parents, by downplaying the sweet taste (and associated sugar content). Food marketers and manufacturers, for the most part, are not your friends in pursuit of your health maintenance goals. They will prey on our weaknesses and lack of awareness at every chance to turn a profit.

Poptarts for Breakfast? Really?

Fast food companies and the "buffet" mentality have led to a fattening of America to the point where nearly 70% of Americans are overweight. Sugar rich foods lead to the release of a substance called "dopamine" in the area of your brain that involves addictive feelings of pleasure. Dopamine release in this same part of your brain is involved in the addictive properties crack cocaine. Furthermore, dopamine regulation is a large part of the function of many anti-depressant medications. Studies suggest that palatable or "sweet" foods may act as self-medicating for day to day stress and depressed mood.

Unfortunately the manipulation of our minds and our appetite doesn't end with just sugar.

Learn more about diabetes and how to combat it at www.yourgainplan.com

Myth #8: Whole Wheat Is Healthy

Breakfast of Champions? Really? Jump Start your Metabolism? Really? Whole Grain Guaranteed? Do you know what that means? In 2002, the trade organization "Whole Grains Council", put out the Whole Grain Stamp for food packages that lets consumers know how many grams of whole grain are found in a serving of the food. The minimum amount to garner a stamp is 8 grams.

The ingredients for a popular whole wheat cereal. may start with whole grain wheat, but the next 3 ingredients are sugar, salt, and corn syrup. The Whole Grain Stamp says 22g of whole grain. If you read the label the total carbohydrate content is 22g. 4g of that is sugar. Some of that sugar may come from the whole grain, but with sugar and corn syrup as ingredients all of that carbohydrate can't be from the whole grain. Are they intentionally being misleading? Why is the total carbohydrate 22g when the total of fiber, sugars, and other carbohydrate adds up to 23g? Food for thought.

Humans are addicted to wheat, as more than ½ billion tons are produced each year. This is not as much as corn, but 40% of corn grown is for production of ethanol based fuel. Wheat is processed into breads, pastas, cakes, cookies, breakfast cereals, etc. and is even used as a thickening agent in many other food products.

Over the last century wheat has been grown via breeding techniques to provide favorable characteristics to not only wheat farmers, but also to food processors. Breeding a type of

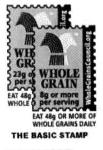

THE BASIC STAMP

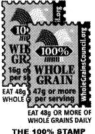

THE 100% STAMP

wheat that is more palatable leading to greater consumption is obviously ideal. How about breeding wheat that contains an addictive substance?

Wheat contains protein in the form of wheat gluten. Wheat gluten has a protein fraction called gliadin. Gliadin is a protein that has some disturbing effects. A study performed way back in 1984 made an interesting discovery. They found that the gliadin fraction of gluten exhibited remarkably high opioid-like activity. In other words, gliadin acted like very addictive heroin in the laboratory. This suggests that wheat gluten proteins may be addictive in their own right despite our addiction to sugars. Furthermore, we know that the opioid addiction medication, naltrexone, helps with weight loss. The author of *Wheat Belly*, Dr. William Davis, has suggested that cultivation and breeding of wheat has led to wheat containing these addictive proteins to the advantage of food manufacturers. By producing more addictive wheat, people eat more and manufacturers make greater profits.

What does all this mean for you? Processed foods that contain wheat flour are potentially addictive and can lead to unhealthy food choices that are hard to overcome. A recent push has been made to eliminate gluten from the diet because of potential adverse health effects. These effects are even more evident in a disease where people have significant sensitivity to gluten leading to intolerance and gut distress. Laboratory studies can be performed to determine if you are sensitive to wheat proteins.

Others suggest that wheat proteins can cause "leaky gut syndrome" allowing more allergens and pathogens to get into your system causing a whole host of other problems like autoimmune diseases and inflammation.

I can tell you first hand that wheat and sugars are addicting. As a bodybuilder, part of my preparation for contests involved fairly extreme dieting to become as lean as possible. I employed the technique of using an extremely low carbohydrate diet with sufficient protein and healthy fats to maintain muscle. The first 2 weeks of eliminating carbohydrates like wheat is very mentally challenging. There are constant cravings and even feelings of withdrawal from carbohydrates like extreme appetite, jitteriness, fatigue, and loss of concentration or focus. However, once you get through that brief episode (~2 weeks) energy levels stabilize, focus returns and even improves, and appetite becomes even less.

It is fairly remarkable how well I would feel on a very low carbohydrate diet. Combined with the drive of contest prep the addiction is easier to overcome. Finding that drive in everyday life is a personal challenge for all of us. But I will give you one more benefit of breaking the addiction to wheat. After you have been away from wheat for so long, the slightest bit of it becomes a delicacy. After contest prep I could always taste the sweetness of foods one-hundred fold. For example, a piece of white bread would have the flavor and pleasure of eating cake. In fact, eating a piece of real cake was overwhelming to almost an intolerable level of sweetness. Check with your doctor first, but I think we should all try a brief "very low carb diet" to understand this phenomenon in your own body.

Myth #9: Treat and Repeat

The U.S. healthcare system, although ever changing, still puts less than 10% of its resources toward prevention. Surgeons are incentivized to perform costly surgeries more than to perform non-operative treatments like orthotics and physical therapy. There is a joke in surgeon's circles, "Every patient is worth 3 operations". This is why I like to be an employed physician with a base salary so that I am not driven to operate more just to make a living. I am not distracted by the everyone must have surgery or "there's a pill for that" mentality

Besides the cost of treating a disease, finding one that is more advanced (i.e. Cancer) increases the chance of dire consequences. There's a lot of debate about the cost of campaigning for prevention and paying for screening tests over the cost of just treating the diseases when they arise. There are complex calculations that go into such decision making in the health care system. I have no interest in making those calculations. I want what is best for my patients, and that is prevention over treatment. I would rather help my patient avoid injury and stay healthy than operate on them.

Do you know when some pain is ok and when it is not? Is it normal to hurt around your joints or your muscle after your workouts? With a basic knowledge base you can adapt and avoid the deconditioning that comes with saying, "just take a break". When injuries occur we employ principles like cross-training, biofeedback, and physical modalities. However, prevention is your main focus. Through use of tools like *The G.A.I.N.* Plan APP, ratings of perceived exertion and attitude, you can determine objectively when your physiology is less than optimal and at risk for injury. With this information, you can progress smoothly up the slope of success without lengthy plateaus.

Myth #10: The Magic Pill

See Objective Measures of Progress, Page 110

"Doctor, I have an ear ache."

2000 BC: *"Here, eat this root."*

1000 BC: *"That root is heathen, say this prayer."*

1850 AD: *"That prayer is superstition, drink this potion."*

1940 AD: *"That potion is snake oil, swallow this pill."*

1985 AD: *"That pill is ineffective, take this antibiotic."*

2000 AD: *"That antibiotic is artificial. Here, eat this root!"*

– Source Unknown

The diet pill market is humongous! With our hustle and bustle society everyone wants a quick fix. If someone could give you a pill that would melt all of your fat in a week you'd probably take it. What if someone said it would work but take 10 years off of your life, would you still take it?

A survey done by Dr. Gabe Mirkin, a sports medicine physician, asked, "If I could give you a pill that would make you an Olympic champion and also kill you in a year, would you take it?" He claims that over HALF of respondents said yes!

Pretty scary stuff, right? This just goes to show how people want to succeed and will take the easy way out at almost any cost.

As you go through *The G.A.I.N. Plan,* I hope you realize that the benefits and feelings of accomplishment in pursuing a goal do not come from the end result, but rather the journey getting there. I can tell you from my experience in becoming a national champion in bodybuilding that it was more fun getting there than being there. As I became known in the sport and took 2nd place at the nationals, the year between my 2nd place and 1st place finish was one of the most exciting and driven years in my life. I was a buzz on the internet boards as the man to beat, active in magazines, and the excitement was electrifying. The moment of winning the nationals was definitely a pinnacle, but the aftermath was one of "What now?"

When we take the easy way out, such as taking a magic pill, we become dependent on the pill. The only thing we learned about the process is that we take a pill and we get thinner. Let's say we get the desired result. Now you have no foundation to maintain your new body other than dependency on a pill. Well, just as we discussed earlier, if you give any one thing to the body for too long you will build a tolerance to whatever that is. Even if you throw an invariable form of exercise at your body, your body will become tolerant and stop adapting (i.e. running at 6 mph for 5 miles every day for years). As you will learn more about as we go, variety is important to induce adaptation to your environment. You will build tolerance to your magic pill or your static exercise routine. As a result you will take more pills and risk your health or you will give up on getting in shape.

Don't get me wrong here, not all diet supplements are useless. Many supplements are beneficial in reducing appetite, increasing fat burning, and improving focus. However, without the proper *G.A.I.N. Plan*, these supplements are quite limited in their long-term benefit. Through proper goal setting, attainment, and maintenance you can make any changes to your health and longevity that you want. These changes to your life-style become healthy habits that will last you many years without developing any tolerance. In the end, your sense of accomplishment will be from the process not the product.

The Placebo Effect

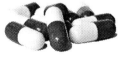

The Placebo Effect can be defined as the response that occurs when an otherwise ineffectual treatment (such as a sugar pill) is given with the pretense that it will have a desired effect and it subsequently does. This effect demonstrates the importance of perception and the role of the brain in controlling bodily functions. The brain controls the processes of pain, motor fatigue, fever, and even the immune system. Functioning of the immune system is controlled indirectly via the sympathetic and parasympathetic nervous system. Surprisingly, the brain can be conditioned to link a sugar pill with the effect of a drug that suppresses the immune system; further supporting the fact that a positive mental attitude can be linked to staying healthy, understanding that one could think their way into being sick!

The placebo effect is pervasive in medical practice and may even be more pervasive in sports nutritional supplementation. Multiple studies have examined the placebo effect in taking pills and found the effect is larger with more pills, higher price, branding, capsules over tablets, or injections over pills. One study even suggested that adherence to taking a placebo may be associated with a statistical decreased risk of mortality. However, susceptibility to the placebo effect only occurs in approximately 30% of the population. Furthermore, until a placebo is tried, we can't predict who will be susceptible to the placebo effect. The effect seems to be more prevalent in treatments expected to improve perceived exertion, fatigue, and pain.

Mind Over Medicine: Placebo Effects
• Pain can decrease in ½ as much as aspirin or even morphine
• Only works if the patient believes it will
• Can increase pain or decrease pain depending on belief of effect
• Bigger pills more effective than smaller ones
• 2 pills at once better than twice a day
• Injection more effective than capsule which is more effective than pill
• Brand names and expensive pills are more effective than cheap ones
• Blue pills work better as downers
• Red pills work better as uppers
• Adherence to placebo pill can decrease mortality
• You can become addicted with withdrawal symptoms from a placebo!

"Placebo controlled" studies are relied on by the Food and Drug Administration to approve the marketing of drugs for treatment of diseases. These are studies where a placebo is given to one group and the treatment medication to the other, but the subjects and the scientists are both blinded to who received which (Randomized Double Blinded Placebo Controlled Study). If the drug performs statistically better than the placebo it is said to be efficacious. If not, any of the effects noticed in the study may be due to the placebo effect. Unfortunately, sports supplements are not held to the same level of scrutiny as drugs. Thus, we need to educate ourselves on which nutritional supplements or training interventions have good evidence supporting their efficacy with placebo controlled trials.

Later in the book I will go over supplements that are backed by science and placebo controlled studies. Much of what I will recommend will be based on the highest levels of scientific evidence as possible.

Myth #11: Fad Programs

Just like diets, there are many distracting fitness and exercise programs out there. 8,7,6 minute abs? Definitely a distraction. However, popular programs have many different exercises and frequently change the volume and intensity. These programs do something that I like: constant change and variety to trick the body into continual adaptation to its environment. However, these programs in themselves are built around a mass audience and don't really individualize the lifestyle or incorporate the other 3 pillars of *G.A.I.N.*, they basically focus on "G". That is not to say they don't have dietary preferences or recommendations, but these are secondary to their exercise routines. In fact, "Uncle Pukie and Uncle Rhabdo" of Crossfit point out the need for the "I" of *G.A.I.N.*, integrated medicine. If you are unfamiliar with these icons of Crossfit, they are clowns that represent the common effects of an excessive Crossfit workout; Puking and Rhadomyolysis (life-threatening breakdown of muscle). If you have medical problems such as chronic injuries, arthritis, or restrictive body fat, many of the movements in these routines can be not only intimidating, but debilitating if attempted.

These programs are for those who desire to achieve or already have a high level athletic performance. These exercise programs are intimidating and dangerous for many others. Although some of these programs scale down for beginners, the end goal is always peak performance at physically challenging and sometimes dangerous exercises. I personally like Crossfit in principle with its treatment of exercise as a competitive event. However, the lack of rigid attention to technique and risk of injury is high. Olympic weightlifting wasn't created to be done for speed at multiple repetitions. Deadlifting should never be done for speed. If you are a healthy risk taker, have at it; but be cautious.

Attention to all of the pillars of *G.A.I.N.* is need for long-term success. All exercise programs should be individualized based on where you are starting from with an emphasis on objective measures of progress and health. By listening closely to your body an individualized program will increase your longevity in the gym and in life.

One of the most difficult aspects of any program is sticking to it. This takes attitude training and goal setting skills. It is very easy to become discouraged with your training. Developing a negative outlook and an inability to objectively measure your progress leads to failure. Objective measures of your attitude and exercising your mind are critical tasks for success in any sport or performance endeavor. *The G.A.I.N. Plan* tackles the underappreciated Body-Mind-Body (BMB) connection which is often neglected in uni- or bi-dimensional programs. On the other hand, holistic programs like Yoga, Pilates, etc. bring in the mindfulness component for control of your body and stress, but lack concrete measures of progress.

Myth #12: The Diet Conundrum

There are so many different "diet" programs out there that it is quite nauseating to try and research it. A new diet program ends up on the internet or news every day. Diet gurus and pseudo-personal trainers are all over the bodybuilding and fitness boards. They always promote dieting for show prep and make drastic changes in your lifestyle for brief 12 weeks at a time. Only, the rebound can be devastating.

"Dieting" vs. Diet

Your "diet" is all the food you consume on a daily basis. "Dieting" is a method of temporarily adjusting your diet with a caloric deficit to lose weight. This can involve a restriction of calories, a change in the macronutrient profile (i.e. low carbs), inclusion or exclusion of certain types of food (i.e vegetarian), or changes in the way that

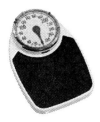

you eat (fast, slow, standing, sitting, you name it , it has been suggested).

The common thread among all weight loss diets is that they all work because of a caloric deficit. However, the majority fail because they are temporary, or unsustainable. It is almost implied that when someone talks of dieting that a diet is something you start and then you eventually stop. Society has been tricked into a belief system that you can go on a diet and get fit and then go off and stay fit. Even though there are more diet programs in the US than ever before, the rate of obesity and associated diseases continues to rise.

In order to overcome this we need a permeating understanding that diet is an inherent part of your life and must be maintained just like your teeth, your cleanliness, and your mind. Societal pressures make this a very difficult proposition. Everywhere you turn there are advertisements for or easy access to fast foods and processed treats. When you see a commercial for fast food and they show a basket of chicken nuggets, fries and an ice cold coke you're taught to think that this is what a meal consists of...really? It is scary to think that when a child sees that, they may believe that they are being told the definition of a meal is; pink slime is a meal? Tackling this problem of pandemic proportions may be beyond the immediate scope of *The G.A.I.N. Plan*, but if you learn to grasp the concept of diet as a way of life, you will be part of the solution.

One of the biggest mistakes people make when embarking on one of these diet programs is that they do too much too quickly and try to starve the fat off. They might see rapid results at first, but they are soon disappointed in their progress or regression. The problem does not arise from a lack of will power, but from deeply rooted evolutionary survival mechanism against starvation.

Ghrelin and Leptin

Research published in the New England Journal of Medicine supports that changes in hormone levels make it very difficult to continue in such diets that have significant caloric restriction. Researchers measured hormone levels in 50 overweight or obese people who had caloric restriction for 10 weeks. The hormones ghrelin (turns on hunger) and leptin (turns off hunger) were measured before the diet, after the diet was completed, and then 62 weeks later. For up to 1 year after the weight loss there were increases in ghrelin (hunger) and decreases in leptin. The signals of hunger were enhanced for up to a year even after a short dietary intervention. This provides a good explanation for why the majority of dieters regain their lost weight within five years.

Dieting and the Brain

Animal research further shows that dieting makes the brain more sensitive to stress and the rewards of high-fat, high-calorie treats. These brain changes last long after the diet is over and encourage otherwise healthy animals to binge eat under pressure. Stress encourages bad eating and makes bad foods more addicting. When you lose a lot of weight on a low calorie starvation type of diet the stress creates long term changes in your brain that make you desire unhealthy foods. Furthermore, you lose more valuable muscle on this type of diet. Later in the book we will discuss how your muscle produces a hormone-like factor that can actually make you smarter! You really have to change the way you eat permanently, but combine it with a comprehensive program of lifestyle changes; including stress management. Return to old habits and the weight will pile on again, perhaps even faster than before.

Yo-Yo of "Skinny Fat"

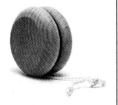

Part of the problem with going on and off diets is the effect that these diets have on body composition. When you diet with a caloric deficit, not only do you lose fat but you also lose muscle. Having more muscle helps you burn more calories and boosts your basal metabolic rate (the energy you burn even at rest, BMR). In other words, muscle is metabolic currency. The more you have, the more you burn. In fact, knowing your body fat percentage can help you to better estimate your daily caloric needs by knowing how much muscle mass you actually have. (See Katch McArdle Formula)

If you are sedentary when dieting, you may weigh less but you also have less lean muscle mass for maintenance of your BMR. Then you fall off the diet into bad habits and you gain the weight back. Only this time your weight consists of a higher percentage of body fat than where you began. Now you decide to try and lose weight again by going on another restrictive diet. Not only is it harder to lose weight because you have less lean muscle and a lower metabolic rate, but when you do lose weight you lose more muscle. The cycle perpetuates itself and you get stuck in a Yo-Yo dieting rut. If anything you can become "skinny fat"– a person who is thin with no muscle.

If dieting was as easy as just taking in fewer calories than burned, everyone could be successful. When you have a daily caloric deficit of 500 calories, it would take 7 days to lose a pound of fat. If you weighed 150 pounds after 50 weeks you would weigh 100 lbs, right? No, probably not. Just as if you were forced to live on 1/3 of your salary you would adjust your budget and spending such that you don't go bankrupt. If your body didn't adjust to the deficits, it would consume itself into a pathologic emaciated state. With extended restrictions your BMR decreases as your thyroid hormone decreases, anabolic hormones like testosterone or estrogen decrease, and your fat goes into storage mode. The fat gets locked down and it is harder to get out.

Below I will summarize how to avoid being distracted by "diet" programs. This applies to any of your goals whether losing weight, winning a bodybuilding show, or getting in shape for a sport:

1. Make your food a healthy habit instead of "diet"

2. Save your muscle with protein and weight training

3. Make any caloric deficit small and shoot for long-term health GAINs

4. Let exercise burn the fat rather than trying to starve the fat

5. Eat more frequently and never skip meals

6. Don't stay in any negative calorie balance for long – Blow on the coals now and then with fuel for metabolism

The emotional aspect of dieting must also be addressed and often isn't. People don't succeed on diets for one of three emotional reasons:

1. They overeat because they're afraid of their feelings.
2. They overeat to reward themselves when they're frustrated or unfulfilled.
3. They overeat to assert their independence, to feel safe, or to fill emptiness.

Next time you catch yourself sitting down with a bag of chips or a big bowl of ice-cream, ask yourself if you are feeding your feelings or fears. Do you feel like the junk food is giving you comfort from your stress? In the long run, the stress will catch up with you and your health will suffer. Be aware of why you eat a certain way.

Write down a diary of when and where you eat for a week. Look for trends like, "I visit my friend's desk at work every day around 3pm. She always has chocolates and I eat a few at each visit." You're escaping the stress and monotony of work. Next time, grab a handful of nuts and munch on them while you're chatting. Keep your hands busy so that you don't reach for the chocolates. Some people have such deeply rooted emotional issues surrounding food that they may need professional help. Don't be afraid to ask your doctor or a counselor to help you lose weight.

The G.A.I.N. Plan Mentality

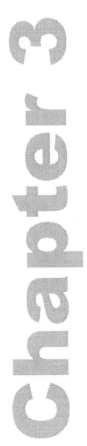

1. Body-Mind-Body Connection

"Humor is nothing but extreme positive thinking."
                                        −R.C. Fields

Unfortunately, we live in a very serious world. When we are infants we laugh hundreds of times per day. As adults we laugh only 1-2 times per day. It is really undeniable that laughing and smiling just make us feel better. Try it right now. Put a smile on your face for 1 whole minute... hold hit really big. It might feel silly, but just try it. Now try not to laugh... read this:

Mahatma Gandhi, as most know, walked barefoot most of the time, which produced an impressive set of calluses on his feet. He also ate very little, which made him rather frail and with his odd diet, he suffered from bad breath. This made him (say it out loud): *a super-calloused fragile mystic hexed by halitosis.*

Feel better already? OK, I'm not a great comedian.

Adding humor to your life is critical to refreshing your mind. I always feel better after telling a joke, as just making people laugh has the same effect on me. I keep a few good ones in the back of my mind and bring them out almost as often as breaking into spontaneous dance.

There's a lot of talk about the "mind−body" connection in modern scientific and contemporary literature. Positive mental attitude and stress relieving strategies like meditation, mindfulness, and even humor can clearly affect your body's physiology. Lowering levels of stress hormones through these techniques has extremely beneficial effects on your health and longevity as we will elaborate on later.

In the medical community we know that pain conditions like fibromyalgia and osteoarthritis share common pathways with depression and anxiety. Medications used to treat these psychiatric conditions, like Cymbalta, can improve pain symptoms and quality of life. Furthermore, the link between the mind and your body's physiology, especially hormones, supports the use of psychological therapy in the treatment of symptoms related to hormonal changes with aging. Science actually supports improving your mind to improve your body and vice versa.

Something that is way too under-recognized is the effect of the body on the brain. It is quite intuitive that if your body is healthy you're probably in a better state of mind than if you were ill and laying in a hospital bed. However, the interplay between your body and mind are very intricate and research is discovering new pathways for the body to manipulate the health of your brain.

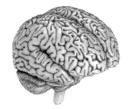

The brain is very "plastic", meaning it is able to grow and make new connections between brain cells (neurons) when it is trained to do so, even as we age. In the area of the brain called the hippocampus, memories and new tasks are learned via not only new connections between brain cells, but also through a process called "neurogenesis"; the growth of new brain cells. Research by Pereira and colleagues (Proc Natl Acad Sci U S A. 2007 Mar 27;104(13):5638-43), has examined how exercise affects this area of the brain. They discovered that exercise was a critical factor in promoting the growth and survival of new cells in the hippocampus. The conclusion that can be drawn is research is: *exercising the body exercises the brain.*

There is belief in the scientific community that the human mind evolved in response to physical activity. In early man, the more "athletic" were those who were more likely to survive. Those with better ability to hunt down their prey with greater speed and endurance did not starve and thus were able to pass down their genes through mating. Evidence suggests that species of animals with large brain sizes relative to their bodies have greater capacity for endurance exercise. However, what came first, improvement in the brain and then performance, or vice versa?

Dr. David Raichlen an anthropologist at the University of Arizona published an article in the Proceedings of the Royal Society Biology (Proc Biol Sci. 2013 Jan 7;280:1750) suggesting that physical activity may have contributed to development of the mind in early humans. Multiple animal studies show that physical activity increases the growth of brain cells in the memory and thought processing centers of the brain. Even studies of children show that increased levels of physical activity correlate to higher intelligence. This probably doesn't include kids who experience brain injury in contact sports like football. I digress. Nevertheless, this carries into young adults and the elderly, clearly correlating physical fitness to better brain function.

One of the more interesting aspects of this research is the finding that growth factors (small proteins that affect cells in the body like hormones) such as BDNF (brain derived neurotrophic factor) can be produced by growing muscle cells (Mol Biol Cell. 2010 Jul 1;21(13):2182-90). BDNF is a protein that muscle releases into circulation. It then crosses the blood-brain barrier and stimulates the formation of new brain cells. This is strong evidence for how exercise stimulates brain development.

So what is all of this telling us? We need to nourish both the body and mind. Whether it is by exercising, meditating, or going to a comedy club there is an undeniable and often underappreciated effect on your health. I know too many people, including myself, who do not take advantage of the stress relieving effects of fun social interactions on a regular basis.

Over the years, I was so focused on success in athletics and school that I put more stress on myself by not letting my brain recuperate. I used to think that if I took a "me time" break with friends or a funny movie that I wasn't being "productive". In reality, I was being more destructive to my body, mind, and friends. My social interactions in my professional swing dancing were the best stress relief a medical student could have.

The G.A.I.N. Plan emphasizes the importance of "active rest" whether it is in the form of relative rest of a body part that is having pain, or actively meditating to refresh your mind. I emphasize the concepts for building and maintaining muscle to not only look better or be stronger, but also to build your brain. Reading this book should be an active escape for you while resting your body after a stressful day. Remember, it doesn't have to happen all at once. Eat the elephant one piece at a time...

Now go to Google and put in "jokes". Find a favorite one to share with your friends and colleagues (relatively clean with a little bit of dirtiness goes a long way over raunchy).

2. Making Successful Change: Turn Dreams into Goals.

"A dream becomes a goal when you give it a deadline." – Unknown

I wrote this book to help you make healthy changes in your life and attain your goals. I believe this can be done while finding new avenues for harnessing your latent competitive spirit to be better than your yesterday's self. Making deliberate change in your life is what creates wisdom. Change presents learning something new and mistakes along the way are inevitable. We learn from mistakes and grow from them. Challenges will arise, and you will rise to the top with the right tools. If you embark on a journey toward a new goal without a map your chances of immediate success exponentially diminish.

I would recommend reading the book, *"Who Moved My Cheese?"*, by Spencer Johnson. You will learn about the mice Hem and Haw who end up stuck in a rut because they became complacent with mediocrity and dependence; like being stuck in a dead end job. It is very

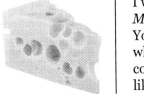

scary to quit that job not knowing if the grass is greener elsewhere. It may not be, but you'll never know unless you try. You may be afraid to look for another job for fear that your boss might find out. However, you may be missing out on the potential advantages of beginning the search. If your boss finds out they may do one of 4 things: 1) fire you on the spot, 2) offer you a raise to stay, 3) realize that you are unhappy and make changes to your benefit, or 4) help you find a job that is more suitable to your needs and interests. Either way, you will be in a better place. Being fired would be scary, but it may just open a new door to new opportunities.

I recall when Iowa State dropped my gymnastics team. It was a complete surprise. I joined Tae Kwon Do to fill the competitive void in my life. Although I competed well and moved up the ranks quickly, I couldn't stand the pain of kicking people in the elbows. My interest in Tae Kwon Do fizzled and my interest in gymnastics was revived. Although I had focused much of my energies on my class work and research in preparation for medical school, I had to be creative to do gymnastics again. I still had desire to be a national still rings champion, but there were no rings at Iowa State. I built a small ring tower in my dorm room and traveled to Chicago to train on weekends. I built great strength on the rings and this was recognized by the Michigan State University coaches. With a "map" charted between my M.S.U. coach and I, I went to the NCAA Championships ranked #1 for the season on the rings.

Looking back it almost seems like this was just meant to be; Academy →I.S.U. →M.S.U.

The experience I gained helped me to accept change and to realize when change is really needed. The stress of change always feels the same as when I was 19, but the process is better planned. Don't be afraid when someone moves your cheese. Go forward and find YOUR cheese! Don't wait for the right time, the time is now.

Goal Setting is a Skill

The reason why *The G.A.I.N. Plan* works is that it focuses on multiple components of goal attainment with orientation toward a healthy wellbeing; it incorporates exercise, attitude, medicine, and nutrition. Setting appropriate immediate, short-term, and long-term goals is critical to success in your *G.A.I.N. Plan.*

"The greater danger for most of us is not that our aim is too high and we miss it, it is that it is too low and we reach it." – Michelangelo

Although setting goals is a reasonably easy process, most of us don't know where to begin. You could just sit down and start writing down your goals. If you haven't tried this, you'll learn that putting a goal on paper requires the patience of "eating an elephant". If you start with a big idea, you're going to have to learn to break it down into manageable pieces. Nothing is more crippling than setting a goal that you can't visualize happening. What Michelangelo is suggesting to me is that we often underestimate our own abilities to achieve greatness. He is not suggesting that we set lofty goals that would be inconceivable to achieve. I believe he is suggesting that we need to have faith that we can accept the challenges faced with change and step out of our comfort zones. He realized that humans learn and grow even when they fall short of their dreams.

Our goals are like our muscles. If we build them to lift a certain weight, we will never lift more weight unless we push them to adapt to a heavier weight. This causes muscle soreness that we can't be afraid to experience. Goal achievement requires stepping out of your comfort zone and adapting to change; LIVE SORE!

It is always amazing to me how many people have never sat down for 30 minutes and brainstormed their goals on a piece of paper. It could be as simple as writing things that you are going to do that day, or as complex as your life-long dreams and aspirations. Most people spend more time making grocery lists, studying, partying, socializing etc. than they ever have at examining their goals for personal growth.

Where are you starting from? Where are you going? What are some of your goals? Write ONE of them down and turn your ethereal thoughts into written word. Start with just one goal until you get a grasp of the process.

End Goal: _____
(Be specific; give an exact outcome, i.e. 150 lbs)

Starting Point: _____
(i.e. bodyweight 190 lbs)

Smallest Manageable Component of Your Goal: _____
(Be very specific; i.e. 1 lb per week)

Today's Goals: _____
(Assess your actions: i.e. burn 250 kcals in cardio, eat 250 kcal less)

Time Required Each Day: _____
(one hour in the gym; 30 minutes of meal prep)

This Week's Goals: _____
(i.e. lose 1 lb)

This Month's Goals: _____
(i.e. lose 4 lbs)

This Years's Goals: _____
(i.e. reach 150 lb)

Life-Long Goals: _____

_____

_____

(i.e. make sustainable changes to maintain my new weight)

When you set a goal you are essentially putting together an "action plan". Once you have determined that your destination will be rewarding, that goal is the main motivator for keeping you on the road to success, with little accomplishments along the way re-fueling your tank. If you don't truly believe your goal attainment will be rewarding, you may be quick to turn around and go home. You need to be honest with yourself. Write down the pros and cons to attaining your goal and make sure that the destination is really something you desire. If your heart isn't into it and you are doing this for the wrong reasons, you will fail.

Pros of Attaining Your Goal: *(i.e. less joint pain, more energy, keep your skinny jeans)*

_____

_____

_____

Cons of Attaining Your Goal: *(i.e. less going out to bars, less eating out, time spent in gym)*

_____

_____

_____

Just as you need to plan for rest from difficult training in the gym (i.e. 5 days on with 1 day off), you need to plan for rest and setbacks in attaining your goals. You need to step back and try to predict what obstacles you might encounter along the way. Now write down some of the obstacles that you might encounter and how you might overcome them:

Obstacles:	Solutions:
1. _____	_____
_____	_____
2. _____	_____
_____	_____
3. _____	_____
_____	_____

Many people fail when they set out on a journey toward a goal because of a lack of knowing what to do. However, once you learn about the G.A.I.N. diet and exercise recommendation you'll have no trouble choosing goals and starting your journey. A well thought-out action plan will bridge the gap between a dream and a goal.

3. Reprogram the Subconscious

You need a plan for reprogramming the subconscious to end bad habits and start healthy new ones. This is done in two ways:

a. Meditative Introspection

b. Repetition

The subconscious mind controls your habitual behavior. If you lived life by consciously thinking about every activity (i.e. the action of brushing your teeth) you may find this a little mentally exhausting. However, without learning how to manipulate the subconscious it is difficult to overcome your deeply ingrained bad habits (i.e. not going to the sink to brush before bed).

Jon Kabat-Zinn has a body of work that explains the concept of "mindfulness" as a form of meditative introspection. This concept suggests that there is "mental noise" that causes one to lose focus. Mental noise includes thoughts that disrupt our focus by interjecting thoughts of the past or future, not the now and not this moment. We pick up more mental noise over time and as an adult we can end up with pathologically disruptive mental noise. This noise and its thought distortions can lead to symptoms of anxiety and depression. The noise only perpetuates yesterday's self therefore preventing you from recognizing today's self. The noise may even make you perseverate on tomorrow's self; losing track of today.

As kids, we didn't have this disruptive mental noise; we could play for hours without any care about what the world thinks of our imaginations We could focus on our imaginary play worlds. We didn't judge those imaginary thoughts, we just enjoyed the moment. Becoming mindful is a way of regaining focus and reprogramming the subconscious to not let experiences interject judgments into our current situation.

Professor Anthony Goodman described mindfulness meditation in an eloquent way in his lecture series. My interpretation is that mental noise is very much like the way we live today. We can be working on a book and the phone rings, an email pops up, or interesting news comes up on the TV. There are many distractions in our daily life that divert our attention away from the real focus (i.e. writing a book or working out). In the same way thoughts can be judged as disturbing and subsequently divert our thought processes. We end up chasing the disturbing thoughts and we become frustrated and anxious. Very much like if you were sleeping and having a nice dream and then a situation from work pops up. You may then wake up and perseverate on that and have trouble falling back to sleep. Get up, walk around a bit, have a glass of warm milk and get back to the nice dream!

When athletes talk about being "in the zone" they find that space between thoughts and live it! I've been there. On the rings at the NCAA

Championships, there were no thoughts that would deter me from giving the best performance of the year. I had no judgments. I only saw perfection. There were no doubts. It was an amazing place to be. You can find that place with focused meditative introspection. Find the place between thoughts in your own mind. Take some quite time each day and try to focus on that empty space between thoughts. Once you find it, you will be able to place your goals into those spots and *keep the doubt out*!

PMA and Reprogramming the Subconscious with Repetition

Reprogramming the subconscious to attain goals and change habits works in the same way. If you judge your actions too often and allow for distractions the programming becomes jumbled. If you set out on a journey but take multiple detours on top of a detour, you will invariably get lost. You must stay focused until your desire to go another direction supersedes.

The subconscious is trained by repetition. We become what we think and when we think scatter-brained, we become scattered. If we think negative thoughts regularly those thoughts will self-perpetuate and become expressed as actions.

Since the subconscious is re-programmed by repetition, we must focus on repeating positive thoughts. This is where the concept of positive mental attitude or "PMA" becomes so important in goal attainment. You must focus your thoughts on what you want to achieve and not on what you want to avoid. If you tell yourself not to think about being fat, you'll inherently be thinking about being fat. If you think about how good it would feel to be in shape you'll be in a more positive mental place. Repeat the positive thoughts in the empty space that you find between the judgmental thoughts. This takes lots of practice which is plenty of repetition.

One of the more common thoughts that I hear expressed to me in my practice is, "I have hypothyroidism and I can't lose weight!". Meanwhile, they are on thyroid hormone and their levels are completely normal now. In reality, perseverating on the hypothyroidism has led the patient to neglect their activity level and dietary intake. By redirecting them to the positives of proper diet and exercise they are able to accept that their ability to change is in their control.

4. Overcoming Procrastination

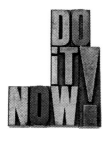

As the saying goes, a dream becomes a goal when you give it a deadline. However, deadlines add stress. Fear of the work ahead or fear of failure leads to procrastination. Procrastination is effectively putting off the inevitable in order to be more comfortable at the present. Unfortunately, as deadlines approach the procrastination compounds the stress through urgency in getting the job done. Often procrastination leads to subpar work and missing deadlines.

Many people feel immobilized by the stress of a deadline. They feel like they need to wait until they are "in the mood" to be productive and accomplish their tasks. They say, "When I'm feeling better I'll be more productive and creative, so I'll just wait."

It is a common misconception that your motivation or desire to work precedes productive action. You may think that you need to be "in the mood" to start working. This misconception is one of the major causes of procrastination. Successful people know that making yourself busy leads to motivation to do more work. If you wait until you feel like doing work, chances are you will never start the work. Taking action in "work", especially in stressful and demanding tasks, is always difficult to do; otherwise it would be called "play". However, the more you do, the more you feel like doing as you see the light at the end of the tunnel. Action begets action... its physics of the universe really. Once you get an object moving, it will stay in motion until it is stopped by an outside force.

Newton's First Law of motion: an object at rest stays at rest or an object in motion stays in motion unless acted upon by an external force. Your dreams and desires need to be the external force to move from rest to motion.

It is important to recognize the stressors associated with achieving a goal. Work will be involved and the process won't always be smooth and straight forward. It's the challenges and obstacles encountered that lead to personal growth, creativity, and intimacy. The sooner you accept that frustrations will be encountered the sooner you will be able to grasp the concept of completing a task. If you have a low tolerance for frustration and require perfection in all that you do, you will be paralyzed by your own expectations of yourself.

Nobody else in the world believes that you will always be perfect, so why would you?

Perfectionism can be a huge precursor to procrastination and the more you procrastinate on a deadline, the more difficult it becomes to make the project perfect! I have suffered from this form of procrastination. It is certainly ok to have high standards in a healthy pursuit of excellence; I certainly do. However, if you base your self-esteem on the idea that everything you do must come out perfect, you will have a significant lack of motivation. Plan to be more motivated by the creative process and the small successes that come with overcoming challenges.

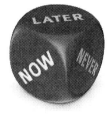

Don't fear failure, as everyone will fail at some point. When success is overly important to your sense of well-being, the fear of failure can be the biggest obstacle to action. Basing your self-esteem on your accomplishments can be self-defeating. Your family and friends will still love you when you have failures. In fact, failures may bring intimacy and comfort from your friends that may not have occurred with successes.

Success can have a few different effects on those around you. First, you may be admired and looked up to for your success. It is important to realize that this isn't "love"; it is an interest in "how'd he do that?" Second, success can lead to jealousy and competition. Many people want fame, fortune, and successful careers in work or sports. People who want what you have may express interest in your accomplishments, but aren't interested in your feelings. It can be a lonely feeling at the top if you put all your interest in your successes. Embrace the challenges and grow from your failures.

Steps for Overcoming Procrastination

If you are procrastinating from doing a task, whether it is finishing a project, going to the gym, losing weight, or preparing for a contest you need to analyze your situation objectively. Here are 5 steps to overcoming procrastination. As you will see, they are very similar to goal setting!

1. **Write Down Exactly What You Are Procrastinating From.**
   Be specific about the task. Avoid overgeneralizing with statements like "I need to start losing weight" and say "I need to lose 10 pounds."

2. **Make a List of The Pros and Cons of Continuing to Procrastinate.**
   It is very easy to see the advantages of procrastinating: you can play more, eat more sweets, go out with friends, etc. However, the cons will take a little more thought and will likely be eye-opening. In this process, you must be honest with yourself as to whether you really have the desire to complete the task.

3. **Build a Doable Action Plan.**
   Make a timeline to start the project, not a timeline to finish the project. If your project has a deadline, be realistic in writing down how long you think it will take to accomplish. You may realize that it will take 30 minutes of your day each day, 5 days per week for 4 weeks. Doing 30 minutes per day during the work week may be easier than trying to find 10 hours in a single day to work on the project. If you make the block of time too

large, it can be a deterrent from your motivation to work. It sounds more painful to have to work for 2 hours vs. a small 30 minute block.

Remember, 1 hour is only 4.2% of your day.

4. **Use PMA.** Identify the negative thoughts that go through your head when you think about completing your task. Are they `reasonable? Would one of your friends think the same way?

Are there cognitive distortions affecting those thoughts? (See ATTITUDE)

By writing your thoughts down, hopefully you will see the self-deception that is leading you to procrastinate. Being positive and realistic will push you forward in doing your action plan. Avoid saying, "I should be doing X" and start saying, "Doing X will be good for me". The word "should" makes you feel guilty and shamed if you procrastinate as if you were breaking a law or doing something immoral.

Are you trying to avoid a conflict? Have you had a fight with someone or are you resentful for something someone said or did? Resent and anger are thought processes that are purely negative. These negative thoughts imprison you from action and lead to passive aggressive behavior. Would it be worth going to jail for 10 years because someone else spoke negatively about you? You say No? Then free yourself from resentment and anger and move on. If that requires that you be the bigger person and apologize first, then certainly do so!

5. Reward Yourself. Just as in goal setting, you need to accept accomplishments no matter how small as a personal success. Even overcoming an obstacle such as recovering from a setback deserves self-recognition for the valuable lesson learned. Instead of insisting that your efforts, "just aren't good enough" or "are too little too late" recognize and embrace the positive. Avoid thought distortions. If you don't think you deserve to be rewarded, write down your concerns and identify the thought distortions.

5. Your Goals and G.A.I.N.

There are 3 goals to which *The G.A.I.N. Plan* plays particular attention: Health Maintenance, Building Muscle, and Burning Fat.

1. Health Maintenance:

a. If you feel that you are at your ideal body weight and you want to maintain that weight while living healthy for longevity, you are trying to maintain. You need to realize that plateaus erode with time. Even though you feel you are at an ideal body weight and in a healthy place, aging catches up with all of us. We need constant change to keep our bodies adapting to the environment. Rolling stones gather no moss. We need to introduce variety in to our diets and exercise or we will fall back.

b. **Upsetting the Applecart: Homeostasis and Health**

Nature and the human body both like efficiency. We call the efficiency and balance of life "homeostasis". Homeostasis is a state of equilibrium that is tightly controlled such that small changes can be easily accommodated for and counter balanced without shutting down the whole system. For instance, the pH of your blood, a measure of acidity, is tightly controlled around a pH of 7.365 by a complex interaction between the GI tract, the kidneys, and various buffers within your body. Blood glucose is also tightly controlled in homeostasis with rises resulting counter measures such as the release of insulin by the pancreas to bring it back down. Blood pressure is tightly controlled by blood vessels, the kidneys, the heart, and many other biological molecules. Body temperature is so tightly controlled that when it goes up significantly, we have no doubt that something has upset the applecart; illness causing a fever.

Nature wants to be efficient at expending energy. It tries to conserve resources as to not overtax your most important organ, your brain. Maintaining muscle requires a lot of energy as the tissue is very biologically active; whereas, fat cells expend very little energy and act to store energy. If you do not use your muscles, you will lose your muscles because the body would find them to be useless consumers of valuable energy. If you don't use it you lose it. It is as efficient as a well-run business. Why pay for a company car that sits in the parking lot all the time? You need to constantly prove to your

body that it needs to keep its muscle
through challenging exercises.

Diseases result from imbalance in your
body's homeostasis. Diseases and
conditions like diabetes, dehydration,
hypoglycemia, hypertension, obesity, gout,
and any disease caused by a toxin are
disruptions of homeostasis. That "toxin"
can be sugar from the food we eat
disturbing pancreatic function, trans-
fats that damage the blood vessel walls,
lack of exercise that weakens muscles
and the heart, UVA rays overpowering
the skin's ability to repair DNA, lack
of sleep overpowering your ability
to stay awake, or even muscle breakdown
products from training damaging your
kidneys. In ideal circumstances,
homeostatic control mechanisms should
prevent imbalances from occurring, but,
in some people, the mechanisms do not
work efficiently enough, are over-depleted,
or the quantity of the toxin exceeds the
levels at which it can be managed. In
these cases, medical intervention is
necessary to restore the balance, or
permanent damage to organs may result.

By recognizing the balance between
stimulus (exercise, dietary changes
and recovery (sleep, stretching, cross-
training, massage, supplements) we can
maximize our efficiency in attaining
our physical and mental goals. Balance
needs to come into play in all aspects
of our lives. Balance between work and
play, exercise and rest, sleeping and

waking, impulse and aversion all lead to well-being. In summary, positive stimuli, like exercise, lead to positive adaptations. Negative stimuli, like smoking, lead to detrimental adaptations. Find your balance. Continue to stimulate change even when you feel lijke you just want to maintain. The body requires constant positive stimulus for change. Otherwise, age-related deterioration will catch up with you. As they say, If you don't use it, you lose it."

Yet I still live by my favorite motto, "Everything in moderation, including moderation". Learning to know when to have a little excess is part of making leaps in accomplishment. (See Functional Over-reaching)

Old Dogs and New Tricks

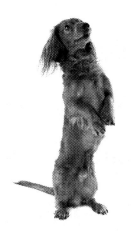

I would like to say that age is just a number in your mind, but when I wake up in the morning at 40 years old with stiff shoulders and knees I am reminded that I'm no longer 20. Does that stop me from occasionally training like a 20 year old? Yes, most of the time. I'm realistic about my physical abilities at my age, but I am not complacent with my level of performance. I know that I can always TRY to improve, no matter how little the results may be. I also realize that if I'm not trying to improve, regression will occur. Complacency will lead to the inevitable decline of aging.

One thing I know for sure is that when I try something new whether it is yoga, running, or swimming I still experience improvements fairly rapidly. Any time you give your body, mind, or muscles a new challenge you will see improvement if the pillars of *G.A.I.N.* are your foundation. You may be surprised that the improvements you make now are even more dramatic than they would've been 20 years ago.

Athletes of all ages and abilities are on a journey to optimum performance and in that quest, age often becomes secondary. Opportunities are more evident now than ever before for older athletes to compete in various sports activities, either within an age bracket "Masters" divisions or in open competition. However, even the most highly-trained athlete will experience a decline in performance after the fourth or fifth decade of life.

If you have been sedentary most of your life or even if you have experienced age related muscle loss, you can improve and gain it back with diet and exercise interventions. To re-iterate, just because studies show that elite level athletic performance decreases with age, this doesn't mean that we can't go from a lower level to a higher level after we have aged. You can still be better than yesterday's self.

It is generally agreed that repeated vigorous activity, including strength training, is extremely important in maintaining robust health into advanced age. Resistance (weights, machines, etc) and balance training improve muscle strength, bone density, and reduce the risk of falling. Even at an elite level of conditioning, the older athlete just needs to be aware that they may need more nutritional interventions and active recovery methods than their younger counterparts. For instance, as we age we become insensitive to the anabolic effects of protein. Studies show that we actually require more protein in our diets with advancing age.

Your parents determine some of your ability to perform both earlier and later in life. If we could only pick our parents we could all be Olympic champions (and millionaires, I suppose). Our genetics can influence up to 50% of our ability to perform at a superior level. However, as we age, the cumulative effect of our environment has a greater effect on our performance level than our genetics.

Maintaining your abilities through the years directly varies according to how much vigorous exercise is performed during later years in life in addition to stress, health, and nutrition.

Stress and Longevity

In theory, stress can affect our longevity by adversely affecting our genes. When our genes are replicated during cell

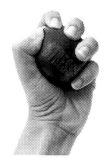

division a little bit of DNA is lost from the ends of the chromosome. To protect the ends, nature has applied redundant DNA at the ends of the chromosomes so that the DNA lost is not DNA important for a coding a particular gene. However, those redundant ends called "telomeres" tend to shorten with each division. Luckily there is an enzyme called telomerase which adds more DNA to the cap. As we age telomerase activity decreases and the important DNA becomes vulnerable to damage as the telomeres shrink. This damage is thought to be a risk factor for generating cancer at the cellular level. There is strong scientific evidence to support that shorter telomeres correlate with higher incidence of cancer. (JAMA. 2010 Jul 7;304(1):69-75)

There are many things that we do in life that can affect telomerase activity. Not surprisingly the more active we are, the better our telomerase works. Exercise of >3 hours of moderate exercise per week correlates with longer telomeres (Menopause. 2012 Oct;19(10):1109-15).

Those with higher levels of cardiorespiratory fitness based on aerobic exercise capacity tend to have longer telomeres protecting their DNA (PLoS One. 2012;7(12):e52769). Conversely, chronic negative physical and mental stress can result in decreases in telomerase activity. Elevated stress hormone levels decrease telomerase activity. Oxidative stressors from our environment like smoking, sugar, and pollution can decrease telomerase activity. Fight the inevitable decline in health by exercising, eating right, and controlling your stress.

Records in endurance events such as running, swimming, and cycling suggest that our physical prime comes during our 20s or early 30s. Although older runners continue to achieve exceptional records for their ages, running performance generally declines with age and the rate of this decline appears to be independent of distance. Studies of elite distance runners where they were followed as they age indicate that despite a high level of training, performance in events from the mile to the marathon declines at a rate of about 1% per year from the age of 27 to 47 years. In a study reviewing American records for both sprints and long runs, performance decreased by about 1% per year from age 25 to 60. After age 60, unfortunately, the records for men slow by nearly 2% per year. Women also show a similar decline in performance. These are consistent findings across studies and many show a more rapid decline per year as we age above 60-70.

Why this occurs could be multifactorial, but the physiology correlates well with decreases in anabolic hormones such as Testosterone, Estrogen, and Growth Hormone. Additionally, cardiac and lung functions decrease with age through decreased responsiveness to hormones.

As a whole, maximal muscle strength peaks between the ages of 25 and 35. Beyond age 35 it is thought that average individuals lose 2% of their muscle strength per year. You are not an average individual; you are a G.A.I.N. Planner! You can prevent this decline with the principles of G.A.I.N.

In sedentary individuals, the ability to stand from a seated position is compromised at age 50 and by age 80, becomes impossible without assistance for many. Another activity of daily living, opening a jar, can be performed by 92% of men and women in the age range of 40 to 60 but after age 60, the failure rate becomes 68% and over 70 only 32% can open the jar. Again, why this occurs is multifactorial and may be contributed by muscle, nerve, hormone, and joint health.

As we age our bodies have reduced ability to mobilize fat from storage for use as energy. Coupled with the loss of lean mass that occurs with decreasing physical activity, body fat percentage can be expected to rise. The amount of body fat in men and women is inversely correlated to their level of physical activity, more so than their diet. In other words, exercising more has a greater effect on being leaner and more muscular than eating better. Strength training exercises have been shown to maintain lean muscle mass better than un-weighted activities like swimming and biking. Moral of the story: Weight training is very important as we age!

Despite decrements that we have described with aging, older athletes are capable of exceptional performances. Their ability to adapt to both endurance and strength training is well-documented. Aging adults may start from a lower baseline when starting a new training regimen but their ability to improve is proportional to that of a younger person's. Older adults even respond greater to resistance exercise when whey protein and essential amino acids are supplemented; more than expected in younger adults.

I think of an older sedentary person as an energy sponge. At first, they are a little shriveled, dried up, and brittle. When you give them the right fuel in the form of nutrition, activity, and social interaction they can expand at unimagined rates becoming flexible and functional.

But returning to the G.A.I.N. Plan theme of gradual progressions, as we age with weaker bones, more brittle tendons, and loss of coordination, we must turn large goals into smaller attainable goals. The body as a whole responds much in the way muscle does to exercise. If you add a little stress (i.e. weight lifting) the homeostasis of that muscle is slightly disturbed and the body brings balance to the system by growing so that is can accommodate that stress later. Nonetheless, if you decide to do too much at once or too much too soon, the muscle either fails under the stress and tears, or it doesn't have time to recover from the previous bout and tears; respectively. As we age we especially need to start low and go slow. As a physician we do this with medications in the elderly. Start with a low dose and slowly increase it so as to not "upset the applecart".

No matter our age, we need to add variety to stimulate change and avoid decline. If you do the same exercises each time you train, eventually that becomes part of your body's equilibrium and it no longer needs to respond by making any improvements. You hit a plateau or worse, go backward. Again, if you don't use it you lose it; keep your mind and body growing by stimulating both with variety in your life. Your *G.A.I.N. Plan* should emphasize gradual improvements by adding gradually increasing stimulus for change.

2. Building Muscle:

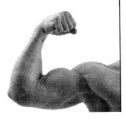

a. For those who want to build muscle, like a physique athlete, *The G.A.I.N. Plan* will give you scientifically proven methods to build lean and powerful muscle.

The G.A.I.N. Plan recognizes that muscle is "Metabolic Currency". Muscle plays a bigger role in your health than just looking good and giving you strength. Muscle is a complex metabolic machine that affects your entire body. The more muscle you have the more metabolic machinery you have to burn fat and maintain the health of other organs like your brain. Remember BDNF from muscle and building new brain cells?

The G.A.I.N. Plan always focuses on maintaining as much muscle as possible, no matter what your goal is. Even those who just want to maintain their health have to fight the inevitable loss of muscle that can occur with aging. For those that want to burn fat, they need to maintain as much muscle as possible to keep their metabolism revved up.

b. Anabolism vs Catabolism

Most of the tissue in your body is constantly remodeling. Many of the cells in your body today are very different than the ones you had 10 years ago. Muscle is one of those tissues that it constantly remodeling and responding to the environment. Muscle responds to stress by adapting. If you lift weights that are heavier than you are used to, the muscle grows stronger. If you run longer than yesterday your muscle gets better at endurance.

Muscle grows via both *Hypertrophy* and *Hyperplasia*. Hypertrophy is the muscle building more muscle proteins that contribute to muscle contraction.

Resistance exercise, like weight lifting, causes muscle hypertrophy. Muscle cells get bigger in size with this muscle protein synthesis. When we discuss "muscle protein synthesis" we are essentially discussing the growth of muscle through hypertrophy. Hyperplasia is where the muscle grows by adding more muscle cells. There are precursor cells called satellite cells that can divide and incorporate more cells into muscle. This is also stimulated by exercise and hormones.

In order for muscle to grow, there must be an anabolic environment. Anabolism is another way of saying building up. Muscle growth is muscle anabolism. The opposite, catabolism, is muscle breakdown. In order for anabolism to occur there must be adequate stimulus (i.e. exercise), anabolic hormones (i.e. testosterone, insulin), and nutrients for growth (i.e. protein/leucine). If any of these factors are diminished, you will not be maximizing muscle growth.

One of the more neglected aspects of the anabolic vs. catabolic cycle is how catabolism is always in balance with anabolism. The goal of exercise, boosting testosterone, and high protein diets is to maximize anabolism. However, there is also a need to limit catabolism. Stress and nutrient deficiencies result in increased catabolic hormones like cortisol which break down muscle proteins. Through stress management, nutritional supplementation, and particular exercise principles presented here in The G.A.I.N. Plan we can minimize muscle breakdown even when burning fat.

3. Fat Burners:

a. These folks desire to lose the extra fat weight while maintaining as much muscle as possible. You may be preparing for a physique competition in pre-contest mode. You might need to make weight for a sport. You may need to lose weight because your doctor told you that you to. Losing weight means that you'll be burning fat and possibly losing some muscle. We want you to focus on burning the fat more than losing actual bodyweight. A proper diet and the right amount of exercise and you will burn the fat.

Fat is a very abundant source of energy in our bodies. Most people have more than 10,000 Calories of stored fat. As we discussed earlier there are two types of fat: White fat and Brown Fat. White fat is the fat that insulates our bodies and acts as storage of excess calories. Brown fat is very metabolically active and contributes to maintaining body temperature, especially when we are young. We want to enhance brown fat activity and burn the white fat stores.

Your body is constantly burning energy stores from the food you eat even when you are sleeping or sitting around. The energy expenditure of your body at rest is your basal metabolic rate (BMR, we will make this synonymous with "resting metabolic rate" for simplicity). This is measured as the number of calories per day your body burns at rest. It can be estimated based on your height, weight, sex, and age. Every activity that you participate in on top of rest adds caloric expenditure to your BMR. If your BMR is 1500 Calories per day, and you perform 500 Calories of exercise your Total Energy Expenditure (TEE) for the day is 2000 Calories.

Although we can estimate BMR through equations based on your body surface area and lean muscle mass, it is important to realize that this is not an exact science. Individuals with the same lean body mass can have vastly different BMRs. One study showed nearly a 30% difference between 2 individuals (Speakman J, et al. Physiological and Biochemical Zoology 2004;77(6): 900–915). This means that when we estimate your dietary caloric needs we have to carefully follow your progress toward your goal. The G.A.I.N. Plan encourages constant "grading" of progress and adjustments as needed.

Your BMR is controlled by hormones released from the hypothalamus and the autonomic nervous system. Thyroid hormone, Epinephrine (adrenalin), and others are important in maintaining BMR. Exercise boosts BMR throughout the day as well as burning fuel during the exercise. Building muscle helps boost BMR by accumulating more "metabolic currency".

Creatine phosphate and Glucose (stored in muscle as glycogen) are the most readily available energy sources for your muscle. If glucose is prevalent, your fat stays in its stores under your skin and in your belly. When you exercise, fast, or go on a low-carb diet and glucose is less available, your body mobilizes fat from its stores to provide a source of energy. Your body burns fat through a process called beta-oxidation. This is the most efficient was your body produces energy. Thus, your body uses this process when you are in an endurance challenge. If you have very low carbohydrate levels, your body will preferentially burn fat throughout the day by converting the stores to ketones (ketosis).

Your brain automatically monitors if there is enough food available as an energy source to keep your BMR up. If you are calorie restricted (as in a low calorie diet) your brain senses this and causes your BMR to decrease to avoid burning up valuable nutrients that keeps the brain functioning. We call this the "starvation response" that kicks the body into storage mode. The principles of *The G.A.I.N. Plan* are intended to avoid ever going into this fat storage mode.

The G.A.I.N. Plan diet is based on a number of scientific principles in order to maximize your lean muscle mass while losing fat or beefing up. The goal of any category above is to stay anabolic and maintain your muscle as "metabolic currency". Losing weight is largely a catabolic process, but anabolic stimuli can still help you to maintain muscle while losing the fat. *The G.A.I.N. Plan* helps you to maintain your muscle by doing a few things:

1. **Teaches techniques to maintain and build muscle through exercise while burning fat.**

2. **Teaches ways to reduce muscle robbing stress.**

3. **Informs you of ways to avoid metabolic dysfunction and injury.**

4. **Gives you an anabolic diet that maximizes your body's ability to maintain and build muscle.**

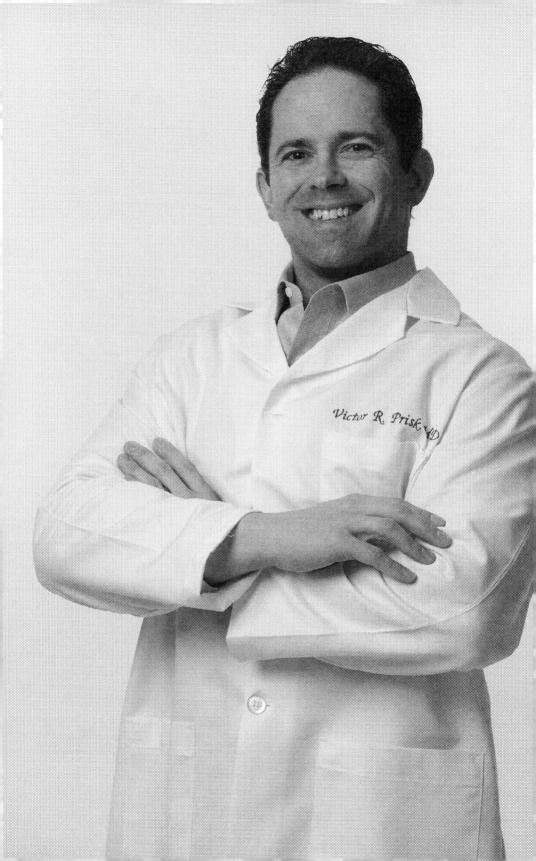

The G.A.I.N. Plan

In the following sections of *The G.A.I.N. Plan*, I will explain the meaning and principles behind the letters of *G.A.I.N.* This will give you an idea of the general principles applied in *The G.A.I.N. Plan* and some of the origins of my recommendations. Keep an open mind and you will see the systematic approach that I take to making healthy change in your life. Of course, the goal here is to "GAIN" knowledge about the way "*G.A.I.N.*" can help you GAIN what you've always wanted... even if you don't currently know what you want.

1. G: Graded Excercise

Since you are reading this book I know you are open to change. The fact that you are reading this book also tells me that you are willing to do a little work to change. With that, you probably know that exercise can't be left out of the equation. You probably have one of the 3 physical goals of building muscle, burning fat, or maintaining health. You may even want to compete in a sport like bodybuilding. For some readers you may already be very active but looking for a new challenge. In your case I want to present you with new creative ways to make you enthusiastic about the gym again. Through harnessing the competitive spirit you will invent a new athlete from within. You may even try taking on the Century Club Challenge.

The Meaning of "Graded Exercise"

The term "graded" exercise has two meanings. First, "graded" means a gradual incline, as in "steep grade ahead". Second, "graded" can refer to receiving an evaluation of your performance,

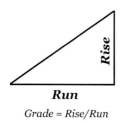

Grade = Rise/Run

as in "the teacher graded the test". Whether you are a professional athlete or a beginner in any activity graded exercise techniques are beneficial in many ways.

Graded = Gradual Incline

In the first iteration of the word "graded", I am referring to a steady and gradual increase in your performance challenges and achievements. One of the hardest things to do in progressing toward a goal is to avoid staying at a plateau for too long. Every exercise program will have plateaus. To say that you can train without ever having a plateau or a setback would be unrealistic. Recognition of the start of a plateau is critical to limiting the length of the plateau and maintaining steady movement forward. Dieters always complain about being stuck at a certain weight. Others just want to break a plateau on an exercise like the bench press. Persistent plateaus lead to disappointment and giving up on your goals. Recognizing the plateau early and changing directions for the better is critical to your progress.

Your goal may be to reach a particular plateau and just stay there. Remember the rolling stone? If you stop for too long the moss will catch up to you. The reality is that plateaus erode with time. When you stop providing stimulus for adaptive changes you end up letting the inevitable decline of aging catch up and your plateau will erode.

Your brain, liver, muscles, heart, and bone are constantly adapting to the environment. The stresses your cells experience determine how they grow. Your cells are constantly turning over and after 10-15 years you are made of almost a completely new set of cells. There is a constant "homeostatic" lifecycle of your cells. When this delicately balanced physiology is disrupted in a good way (i.e. exercise) vs. a bad way (i.e. over-eating) adaptive responses go respectively in one way or the other. Careful disruption of the homeostasis is like taking 2 steps forward and 1 step back. By pushing your body beyond its comfort zone you induce change. However, you must realize that the 1 step back is always a part of the equation.

If you decide that you are going to run a 5K and you have never run before, logic would say that you need to make a very gradual progression towards this goal. If you are overweight and out of shape and you start running 2-3 miles every day without rest, you will go into "recovery debt" and your body will breakdown. This could mean a stress fracture in your foot, tendinitis in your knees, or chronic fatigue. This is when you start sliding down the hill instead of ever reaching your goal.

You should embrace the concept of moving 2 steps forward and 1 step back in all that you do. The sooner you realize that exceeding your limits will result in a need to recover, the sooner you will realize that it is the steps back that make you grow! 5 steps forward can lead to a recovery debt that sends you 6 steps back. This brings us back to the question, "How do you eat an elephant?" Don't bite off more than you can chew. You need to eat the elephant fast enough that the meat doesn't spoil, but not eat so much that you become sick and unable to eat.

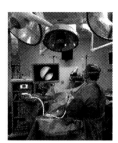

I embrace this in my orthopaedic surgery practice. When you have been off of your foot for 6 weeks because of surgery it is important that you take gradual progressions to getting back on your foot. I explain that the bottom of your foot has lost its durability and you need to build up your "callouses" gradually. If you do too much too soon or too often (The Terrible Too's) it will be like taking 5 steps forward resulting in 6 steps back. Yes, that means you will be expending a lot of forward energy only to go backward. If you create a "blister" on your foot rather than a callous, you could be in so much pain you don't want to walk on it for a while. By taking gradual, steps forward you can achieve forward momentum with 2 steps forward and 1 step back. There is a "just right" or "Goldilocks" zone for everyone. Some may need 3 steps forward to overcome a tendency for 2 steps back. Some may be able to take 1.5 steps forward and get the forward response they need. *The G.A.I.N. Plan* will give you tools to realize when you are doing too little or too much.

This same scenario can be applied to a new running program or weight lifting program. Why run until you are blistering on the first day? Why lift weights to the point that you are sore for a week. You'll just end up taking the rest of the week off to heal. You don't have to push your body to its limits every day. Include variety in your rest and intensity.

The "G" of *The G.A.I.N. Plan* is referring to graded exercise that leads to steady progress with moderate adaptive challenges inserted along the way. These principles can be applied to almost any type of training program, and depending on where you are starting from the intensity level will be specific to you. Make the adaptive challenges in your plan entertaining, invigorating, or inspiring.   Lift with new machines, challenge a friend to a contest, shoot for personal best, push your limits.

Graded = Judging Your Progress

It is really hard to stay motivated without knowing whether or not you are making progress toward your goal. By "grading" yourself along the way it becomes clearer as to whether you are progressing or regressing. By measuring progressions you can compete with your yesterday's self or others while pacing your workouts. *The G.A.I.N. Plan* will provide you with some guidance on how to grade your progress.

Sometimes the goals that led you to use *The G.A.I.N. Plan* may have a subjective basis. For instance, your goal might be to make your body leaner, sleeker, and more aesthetic for performing arts, physique competition, or self-esteem. In that case the mirror can become the judge. However, with the wrong point of view in front of the mirror your attitude and emotions may get in the way. In my personal experience bodybuilders and physique competitors who look in the mirror multiple times per day just can't seem to recognize their own progress. They need an outside point of view or at least an objective measure of progress. It is hard to see the forest when you are staring at a tree.

On the other hand, if your goal is to gain muscle, lower your body fat percentage, run longer, or lift more weight this can be measured objectively. You probably have a scale in your bathroom. Stepping on it at the same time every morning will give you an objective and recordable measure of your changes in weight. But be careful, measuring too often may result in over reacting to normal fluctuations in weight that occur with food intake, fluid balance, and exercise. Body fat percentage is also measurable but there is a great deal of variability in the different measuring options available.

Objective Measures of Progress

1. Body weight (morning, fasted, and after first bathroom)

2. Body fat percentage

3. Resting heart rate

4. Heart rate recovery and variability

5. Strength (i.e. 1 or 10 rep max, number of dips, etc)

6. Speed and endurance

7. Muscle size (circumferential measurements, photo comparisons)

8. Blood Lipids, Hormones, Physical Exam

9. Ratings of perceived exertion for a given exercise intensity

10. Attitude questionnaire

BF% Measuring Tool	Pros	Cons
Calipers	Ease, minimal training required, cheapest tools	Accuracy require consistency in measurement, not useful in very obese, +/- 3 to 5% error
Bio-impedance	Fast, cheap, easy	Hydration status effects number, in altheletes very inaccurate
Bod Pod/DEXA/ Hydrostatic Weighing	Accurate	Expensive, time consuming, lack of availability

The percentage of essential fat is 2–4% in men, and 10–12% in women. This is the minimum amount of fat needed for maintaining body temperature, cushioning organs, and having emergency energy storage.

I also encourage you to integrate general health outcomes into *The G.A.I.N. Plan*, thus the "I" for Integrated Medicine. In the medical world we have many measures of your progress in health. It could be a simple measure such as your resting heart rate or it could be a complex measurement like a graded exercise stress test with VO2max testing. Your physician can follow your lipid profile and give you assessments of your improvements in cardiac risk factors. As a general rule, I recommend routine evaluation by your physician to understand if your goals are helping you to gain health and longevity safely.

The concept of grading yourself will be distributed throughout *The G.A.I.N. Plan*. We recommend following your nutrition objectively. You need to be sure that you are properly fueling your body to progress toward your goal, whether that is to lose weight, gain muscle, and everything in between. Every time you decide to make a new diet or training goal, objectively evaluating your nutritional intake will help you to make finely tuned adjustments to your plan without revamping or loosing track.

Similar techniques can be used to assess your attitude. By using questionnaires and self-assessment techniques, you can enlighten yourself as to how well you are maintaining a positive mental attitude, which is critical to success in any goal. As with any grading, objectivity is the key to accurate assessment. I will give you ways to objectively assess your attitude.

You should always keep your "ego in check". Remember this line from *Top Gun*: "Son, your ego is writing checks your body can't cash". Don't let your ego take you 5 steps forward and 6 steps back. It is a debt that is incredibly painful to pay back.

TRAINING PRINCIPLES FOR G.A.I.N.

In the following section, I would like to give you a summary of the training principles I have always applied to my workouts. I think these principles are essential to the success of your training.

1. Be Father Time: Make Time.

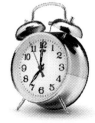

It is very easy to use the excuse that you are too busy to work-out. If you really are too busy, you have not put enough priority on your health. Do you watch TV? Do you spend time on social media? Can you do these while exercising instead? There will be days where there is trauma in your life and working out is just not going to be in the cards. However, if you prioritize your health you will make time to exercise.

It is important that you set a time for how long your workout will be and stick to completing it in a timely and efficient manner. Spending extra time in the gym can lead to burn out and a procrastination mentality. A strength training workout can be done in 30 minutes, high intensity interval training can be done in 15 to 20 minutes, and low intensity steady state cardio 30-60 minutes.

If you know that the end of your day is going to be unpredictable and filled with responsibilities to others (i.e. kids, spouse, pets), then do your workouts before they wake up. This may require a little compromise with your "in-bed" time to get a full 7-8 hours of sleep, but it will be some "me" time when all others are likely snoozing. The early bird gets the worm, right?

If you are only getting 4 or 5 hours per night of sleep you need to re-organize your life. Just remember, your health will help you be more successful for longer in life. As my mentor Dr. Bill Hamilton always said, "Don't be the richest corpse in the graveyard"

Mid-day workouts are possible, but definitely require daily planning and packing of gym clothes. Running the stairs in your office building, jogging around the block, or pushups, sit-ups, and squats in your office can help to make up for days when the gym just won't be feasible. Besides, this is a great time to work on a few of the *Century Club Challenge* exercises.

One of the easiest ways to ensure a workout is to join a gym that is on your way home from work. I pack gym clothes each day and plan to stop at the gym, no matter what. Sometimes you will feel completely exhausted from work and anticipate lying down on your couch. I know this feeling all too well. Avoid the temptation and at least do some cardio and stretch. Just the act of getting on the treadmill or the elliptical will re-vitalize your mind and make you happy that you stopped at the gym for some stress relief. *Remember, action begets action.* Just getting started will motivate you to do more. Break the procrastinator mentality.

If you have been training with high intensity over the course of a couple weeks, the fatigue might be your body telling you that you are overreaching or overtraining. (See Integrated medicine).

You may want to do all of your workouts at home. If so, pick equipment and exercises that will keep you interested. If you buy a piece of exercise equipment, DO NOT let it become a clothing rack! If there is a doubt in your mind as to whether you might use a piece of equipment, don't buy it. Try your equipment out before you buy it and make sure it is something you find comfortable. There is nothing more irritating than an exercise bike that chafes your groin. Cardio equipment comes in all sorts of sizes and durability. Check cardio equipment out at the store first.

2. Actively Rest.

It is critical to recover from your training to avoid the consequences of *"recovery debt"*. When you are training toward a goal it is very easy to think, more is better. You may do 5 straight days of weights and cardio and think it's good to just keep going. In reality it is best to incorporate at least 1 rest day in at most every 5 days. That day can involve relative-rest or complete rest.

Relative rest can include stretching, low intensity steadt-state (LISS) cardio, yoga, message, or just a full spa day. Plan these days as something to look forward to; this day is a way to recharge your mind and your body. One good way to do this is to have a relaxing day riding a bike, going for a walk, playing a recreational (low intensity) sport with friends. Even though you might still be active on these days you are relatively resting with regards to both intensity and focus. Your body is resting and your mind is recovering.

3. Rotate the Tires!

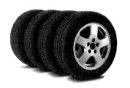

It is important that when you are training toward a goal that you are systematic with your workouts. You can avoid over stressing one body part for too long by changing emphasis regularly. For instance, when I was training to do a routine on the rings, I couldn't just go in and do full routines every day. This would lead to overtraining and possibly overuse injury, as I experienced in high school and early in college. I learned the hard way that I needed to split up days with strength moves and days with swing to recover from all the strength training. I had to add in rest days when I knew that swing or strength would be too much on my shoulders. On those days I would do some tumbling or vault and emphasize leg training.

This can be applied to your body in a weight training routine as well. As an example, if you have a tendency for your shoulders to become sore and painful it is best to space out your shoulder intensive workouts like chest and shoulder training. One way to do this is to space out your routines with either relative rest/cardio or alternate between upper and lower body exercises. One routine might look like this:

SAMPLE ROUTINE SPLITTING BODY PARTS
- Monday: Chest and Triceps
- Tuesday: Quads and Core
- Wednesday: Back and Biceps
- Thursday: Relative Rest
- Friday: Shoulders and Core
- Saturday: HIIT, Hamstrings and Calves
- Sunday: Relative Rest

This routine splits up the shoulder abusing chest and shoulder days as much as possible while getting in all of your body parts. Additionally, this routine could incorporate variations in number or sets per day and the intensity of the training. For instance, you may want to focus more on triceps doing up to 12 sets versus doing 6 to 9 sets of chest on the weeks where you do a heavier shoulder day.

When you combine body parts in the same workout such as back and biceps, it is good to change the order of exercises and the intensity of each body part. One week you may start with doing all of your biceps exercises before your back exercises. You can go heavy on the biceps that day, but then you'll need to go lighter on back exercises as biceps contribute to the movement. The following week you can switch this around.

4. Adapt to your Goals

It doesn't make sense to do all strength training if your goal is to just lose body fat. Strength training can definitely assist you in losing body fat with a well-planned diet because it maintains muscle mass, your metabolic currency. However, cardiovascular exercise is distinctly better at mobilizing fat stores. So it would make sense that you put some emphasis on cardiovascular training. Conversely, if your goal is to have big biceps don't wait until the end of your workout to target them. Focus your energies on your goals.

FAT-LOSS ROUTINE
- Day 1: Upper body resistance training and LISS Cardio
- Day 2: LISS Cardio
- Day 3: Lower body resistance training
- Day 4: Relative rest; stretching
- Day 5: HIIT
- Day 6: Relative rest; stretching
- Day 7: Core training and LISS Cardio

MUSCLE BUILDING TRAINING ROUTINE:
- Day 1: Chest
- Day 2: Back
- Day 3: Legs
- Day 4: Relative rest; stretching

- Day 5: Shoulders, abs, calves
- Day 6: Biceps and triceps
- Day 7: LISS and core exercises or weak body part

LOSING FAT AND GAINING MUSCLE

- If you want to gain muscle and gain endurance, consider a continuum of circuit based weight training while maintaining a heart rate in the cardio training zone of >70% of your HRmax.

- If time is no object for your goals, you can consider doing morning cardio and weights later in the day. Morning fasted cardio is useful in mobilizing fat stores.

- If you don't have time to do 2 workouts, cardio can be done before, during, or after your weight training.

  - If you plan to lift heavy it doesn't make sense to exhaust yourself with cardio first. You could do some low intensity cardio for 10 minutes to warm-up your muscles, but the majority of the cardio can be done AFTER heavy lifting.

  - If your weight training is at lower intensity doing cardio before, in the middle of, or after your weights is reasonable and science doesn't support one over the other. However, recent animal data suggests that the muscle growth stimulus is greatest when weight training is performed after cardio. In fact, the stimulus is even greater up to 6 hours after the workout session.

ADJUST YOUR REPS TO YOUR GOALS

- One frequently asked question I get is, "How many reps do I do for building muscle?" Here are some guidelines for goals and their rep ranges (exhausted movement in last rep):

  - Building Strength: 3-6 reps
  - Building Muscle: 8-12 reps
  - Building Endurance: >15

- It is not realistic to think that if you squat 40 lbs for 100 reps that you're going to be able to increase your squat strength on a single rep max. It is also reasonable to believe that 1 rep maxing is not going to provide the "time under tension" or exercise volume necessary to build muscle. When you train, keep your volume and intensity in alignment with your goals.

5. Know What Your Body Can Handle!

It is very easy to embark on the wrong exercise plan without adequate guidance. If you start an exercise routine with the wrong exercises, intensity, or duration you may be "sorely" disappointed. Excessive soreness, especially around joints, following a particular type of exercise often means you did a little too much too soon.

It is probably intuitive that if you have knee arthritis running and impact activities won't be the best for longevity of your knees. However, some people just don't realize that the constant pounding can be causing further damage thus accelerating the joint degeneration. Sometimes it is less obvious as to when an exercise might be inappropriate.

For instance, you may be 20 lbs overweight and decide to start up on a running program. Your friend tells you that there is this new way of running that is supposed to be natural and more like running barefoot in minimalistic shoes. So you buy the minimalistic shoes and embark on your quest to run a 5K. Next thing you know, you have constant pain in your foot with walking. Your foot is so swollen and painful that you can't even think about running. When you finally get an X-ray, you find out you have a stress fracture. What has happened is that your extra 20lbs which correlates to an extra 60 on your feet (>3x bodyweight loading occurs with running) is now adding stress to bones that weren't accustomed to the impact. Your bones acquired recovery debt to the point of bankruptcy. Add unsupportive running shoes with poor technique and you have a recipe for a stress fracture.

This is where you must integrate medicine and graded exercise. When deciding on an exercise you need to work around your physical limitations. Your physician or physical therapist can help you define your limitations.

If you are a weight lifter and you are looking to become more heart healthy, you may experience some difficulty in the transition. One thing to keep in mind is your weight. The bodybuilder who is 5 foot 9 inches and 230lbs may not want to engage in running as this would lead to incredible stress on the knees. The elliptical, bike, or step-mill may be better options for the larger bodybuilder. If you have a treadmill gradually inclining the grade while walking at 3-4 mph may be an effective way to get your heart rate into the training zone of 65-85% HRmax. Performing pyramids or interval training using the incline or tension on a cardio machine can be a very effective way to get a training effect without adding impact to your joints.

6. Variety is Fuel for the Body and Mind!

One of the problems of many cookie cutter one-dimensional programs is that there is a lack of variety that can lead to boredom and stagnation. Muscles become accustomed to particular exercises just as you can become accustomed to living in different altitudes.

When you move to a different altitude (i.e. into the mountains of Colorado from the plains of Illinois), your body adapts by producing more oxygen carrying red blood cells. When you train your muscle it adapts by building more contractile proteins and recruiting new oxygen carrying blood vessels to the muscle. If you spend too much time doing the same routine without changing the intensity, volume, or exercise type, your body stops adapting. That's when it's time to change your altitude and attitude; kick it up a notch.

Changing things up can be as simple as changing the order of your weight lifting exercises. On leg day, if you always do squat→lunges→deads →extensions→curls, try reversing the order on your next leg day. You may find that doing your squats with more fatigue allows you to lower the weight, concentrate on form, and still get the stimulating effect of exhaustion at 8-10 reps. You could also do this more randomly.

To apply variety to the *Century Club Challenge*, you could make a set of 10 index cards with one of the exercises listed on each card. Shuffle the deck of cards and pick a card until all the exercises are done. Likewise, you could make a list of your 10 favorite back routine exercises on index cards. Pick 4 or 5 cards at random and do those exercises on your back day.

One of the biggest complaints about endurance and cardio training is that it is too boring. Sitting on a bike and going at one pace for 45 minutes can definitely get boring. If you want to make time go by quicker there are a number of things you can do.

First of all, some types of cardio equipment have preset interval/mountain/random routines that can make the intensity of the training go up and down by altering either the incline or the tension. Second, you can occupy yourself with mind games, meditation, or reading. This is only really possible in low intensity steady state cardio. Third, you can change it up by changing the direction of your pedaling or walking by alternating between forward and backwards. Fourth, you can set time, heart rate, or distance goals throughout the workout.

One fun way is to look at the clock and challenge yourself to a distance or step number goal in a certain amount of time i.e. try to complete 100 steps on the stepper before the next minute is up. This will get you to increase the intensity while breaking the boredom.

Finally, you can train with a partner or partners. Partners who have competitive spirit will make workouts more enjoyable. A partner may also recommend exercises you've never tried before.

7. Shock The System!

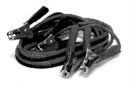

As we just mentioned, you need to shock the system into adapting to its environment in order to reach maximal performance enhancement. You can do this by confusing the muscle with new exercises, different rep ranges, and different order of exercises. Otherwise, your workout intensity needs to reach a level that is going to shock the system into adaptation. This is not to say that an entire 60min workout should be done at an intensity to shock the system. Workouts should consist of an adequate (5-10min) warm-up, working sets, high intensity sets, and a cool down/stretching. So how do you know you have "shocked the system"? There are a number of measures:

a. RATING OF PERCEIVED EXERTION

    Using an RPE scale, you can determine whether you have reached a high enough level of intensity. With "0" being complete rest and relaxation and "10" being on the verge of passing out from over-exertion a level of 8-9 is required to induce change.

b. SETS TO FATIGUE/FAILURE

    If you are lifting weights, pick a weight that leads to failure of the lift at your desired rep range. If you are training to failure to keep your intensity up, you should plan to have a partner to spot you on heavier lifts (i.e. Bench or Squat). One way to boost your intensity is to incorporate "drop sets" or assisted reps at the point of near failure. (See the Weider Principles)

c. HEART RATE

Using the *G.A.I.N. Plan* Monitor you can assess whether you are hitting your desired heart rate intensity. In order to get a good training effect it is important to see a significant rise in your heart rate. High intensity training should bring your heart rate to >85% of your HR_{max}.

d. ARE YOU SWEATING?

Believe it or not, just the act of sweating tells us that we are working pretty hard. This isn't very accurate and can be hard to measure in dry climates, but it does tell us that we are working. This really is a component of perceived exertion.

"Sweat is fat crying!"

e. ENHANCING TRAINING INTENSITY (Weider Principles)

I have adopted many of the principles that Joe Weider proposed in his magazines over the years. I have put them in my own words here.

• *Pyramid Sets*:

Performing your sets in a pyramid with increasing and then decreasing intensity allows for warm-up and muscle familiarity with an exercise before hitting the working weight. If your goal is to do 8 hard reps at 100 lbs, start with a set of 50lbs for 15 reps, then 75 lbs for 12 reps, then do 2 working sets of 100 lb for 6-8 reps, and finally drop the weight back to 75 lbs for 8 reps-10 reps. The less rest you take between sets the more intense the pyramid set becomes. For a very intense workout this can be done as one "giant set" with 3-4 climbing sets and 3-4 dropping sets.

- *Drop Sets*:

Drop sets can be great for increasing time under tension, muscle growth, and muscle endurance. This involves starting with sets at a heavy weight and decreasing the weight at the time of failure to a lighter weight to do more sets:

100 lb for 6reps→Failure→75 lb for 4-6rep→Failure→50 lb for 4-6reps→Failure

If your goal is to do 100lbs for 8 reps and you can only do 6, the drop set will condition your muscle to work through the fatigue barrier. Your muscle will become more accustomed to the "burn" of lactic acid and your endurance with a particular weight will improve quickly. The next time you train go for 1 more rep with the same starting weight!

- *Supersets*:

Supersets are often done with two exercises done with little to no rest between each exercise. The goal with this technique is to step up the intensity and volume of the workout. This is excellent for producing the "pump" and increasing the muscle's time under tension. There are 3 ways that this is often done:

1. Combining opposite muscle groups (i.e. bicep curls and tricep pushdowns)

2. Combining a compound movement with a specific movement (i.e. Squat and leg extensions, standing barbell curl with concentration curls)

3. Combining a heavy movement with a lighter one (i.e. bench press and pushups)

Circuit Training is similar to a superset with 3-5 exercises that can be done in sequence without any rest between sets. Circuit training becomes a "giant set" when done to exhaustion after the last exercise and rest is employed before the next set of the circuit.

- *Cheat Reps/Forced Assisted Reps*:

When you reach failure/fatigue in an exercise, sometimes pushing through a few more reps with some assistance or "cheating" the movement can stimulate adaptations to build strength and endurance. The best way to do this is with a partner who can assist you through a few more reps by spotting the weight. This takes confidence in your training partner and experience working together. The better your partner knows your limitations and how quickly you fatigue with a particular weight, the better they will be at assisting you.

If you do not have a partner, you could do a few "cheat reps". This is a more advanced technique. If you are very familiar with an exercise, you can "cheat" a rep by sacrificing strict form and using momentum to your advantage. That is, you can swing the weight a little or bring other muscle groups into the movement to assist the weight up (often with a bit of a grunt). If done poorly, too often, or with too much weight this can lead to injury and formation of bad habits. The tendency is to bring your back into the movements to swing the weight which can be injurious. Always keep your core muscles (abdominals) tight and use your arms, hips, and legs to assist your movements. For instance, in standing barbell curls don't arch your back to force the weight up. Time the curl with a bend in the knees to assist the weight up, keeping your core tight and upright.

- *Negatives*:

  All movements have a "positive" and a "negative" component. The positive movement is the concentric motion where the muscle is shortening as the weight is being moved (i.e. curling a dumbbell up). The negative movement is the eccentric motion where the muscle is lengthening as the weight is being moved (i.e. lowering the dumbbell down).

"Negatives" or Eccentric exercises are ones that focus on controlling the weight while the muscle is lengthening. For instance, curling a weight up in 1 second and lowering it down in 5 seconds. Sometimes weight can be added to the eccentric movement as this is a very strong contraction. A partner can help with the concentric movement while you slowly lower in the eccentric.

Many studies show that eccentric or Negatives lead to significantly more muscle soreness, but they also lead to a significant muscle growth response. You should always focus on controlling the weight in the negative movement because it is during this lengthening contraction that many tendon injuries occur.

Focusing on this aspect of the movement with moderate weight can be useful for breaking through training plateaus. Knowing that you will have significant muscle soreness the next day, incorporate negatives in a routine with active-relative rest.

- *Super-Slow*

  Super-slow movements are similar to negatives, but the weight is moved slowly in both the concentric and eccentric movement significantly increasing the time under tension. Super slow refers to the time it takes to complete the concentric and eccentric contractions. The concentric or eccentric can be emphasized or done in equal cadence. Slowing the movements down to >5 seconds on the concentric and >5 seconds on the eccentric leads to significant increases in time under tension.

With trial and error, you will realize that when doing this technique you will have to reduce your poundage significantly to reach the same rep range. If you can curl a 100 lb barbell, you may find that this exercise is quite challenging at 50-75 lbs. The slower you go the harder it is, so change it up and try a variety of cadences.

- *100s!*

  This is a technique that the Century Club embraces to its core. Adding a 100 rep set with a weight that you can confidently finish 100 repetitions in one set can be a great way to challenge any muscle group. If you haven't tried this already, you will discover that even a light weight can make you very sore!

  Whether on bench press, barbell curls, military press, squats, leg extensions or lunges, you will discover that getting to 100 reps without stopping leads to an intense workout that will invigorate even the hard-gainer.

  I often employ this technique when I really don't feel like training and I need to get motivated. Reaching the goal of 100 reps with even a light weight gives me a great sense of accomplishment and the burn literally wakes me up. This really becomes a competition between your body and mind. The intense burn and fatigue will test the strongest of wills.

- *Constant Tension*

  This is where you are careful not to "lock" out your joints at the top or bottom of a particular movement. For instance, always keep a slight bend in the knees at the top of a leg press or squat. Just like the super-slow technique this keeps the muscle under tension through more of the movement.

- *"Pump" Training*

  Pump training is focusing on getting a good "pump" in your muscle. The "pump" is fullness in the muscle that makes your skin feel tight and can even lead to stretch marks in extreme cases. Bodybuilders employ this technique in their training as well as before competitions to look bigger on stage. This can be done by employing many of the above techniques. The goal is to get as much blood flow to a particular muscle group before moving on to the next. This can be done with low reps in giant sets or higher reps in supersets. An awesome way to do this is to perform a small circuit of 3-5 exercises focusing on the same body part with no rest between exercises.

  1. The constant contraction of a single muscle group leads to increases in blood flow to that muscle group as well as a decrease in return of the blood from the muscle. Constant contraction of a muscle group can restrict venous blood return. This keeps the energy metabolites in the muscle producing metabolic stimulus for muscle growth and adaptation. Adding isometric contractions to this technique

such as bodybuilding posing can add to the pump. Similarly, you can hold a 2-3 second contraction of the muscle at the top of your exercise, much like doing a bodybuilding pose.

2. Partial reps also bring in this isometric contraction. Partial reps are where you do half of a movement pausing in the middle without going through the full range of motion. This can be employed as "5 position Pushups" or "21's". 5 Position pushups are where you divide a pushup into 5 positions with the top being designated #1 and the bottom (not on the floor) as #5. With a partner you can alternate calling out a particular number, not necessarily in numerical order, and you hold a particular position until a new number is called out. "21's" can be done with any exercise, but is well known as a type of bicep curl. This is where you perform 7 reps of the bottom half of a curl, immediately followed by 7 reps of the top half of a curl, and then performing 7 full repetitions of curls all without putting the weight down. One set of this and your biceps will be on fire with the burn and pumped up minutes later.

You could also use a technique of short pauses after an exercise (i.e. 10 seconds) with immediately continuing with as many reps as possible. This can be done a few times after an exercise and is very effective in stimulating the pump and building endurance with a particular weight. This technique is excellent for improving your ability to get through the Century Club Workout.

It takes practice to recognize when this technique is leading to diminishing return during your workout. After a while, the pump will start to fade, even if you are stil ltraining hard. The goal is to recognize the fade as soon as it starts and move on to the next muscle group.In general, with your body part workouts, when you feel that the blood flow is no longer increasing to the muscle group or even fading you need to move on to the next set of exercises. If you go to the gym and you can't elicit a pump at all, then you need to take a break. A lack of a pump can mean that you are over-trained or under-nourished.

There are many supplements designed to increase this feeling of the pump and are discussed in the "N"utrition section.

- *Progressive Resistance*:

  The goal with any training is to GAIN or at least maintain strength or endurance. Since we can't stop the aging process, we have to keep adding stimulus to our training otherwise the same routine over time will lead to diminishing returns. In every workout you should attempt to lift a little more, go a little harder, or go a little longer—principle of graded exercise—a gradual incline. This is not to say that you need to do this with every exercise with every workout, but you should employ some progression with each workout to be better than yesterday's self.

In order to do this it is very important to avoid over training and be well recovered from your past workout before trying to progress forward. You can increase weight, decrease rest, increase reps, or hold contractions longer. Whichever you do, you are adding adaptive stimulus to your muscle.

- *Pre-Exhaustion*:

  This is a technique used to help limit the amount of weight needed on bigger movements to get an effect. The idea is that you do a targeted exercise such as leg extensions before doing a compound exercise like squats. By working the muscle first, you won't have to lift as much weight to get a stimulus from your bigger movement. This can help prevent added stress on joints or the back by lowering the weight used. This is excellent for working muscle growth, but probably less helpful in adding strength in your squat.

  This technique also gets you to "feel" the pre-exhausted muscle more during the compound movement. For instance, pre-exhausting the quadriceps on leg extensions makes you "feel" the quads more than the glutes or hamstrings during a squat because they are pumped and slightly fatigued.

FAT BURNING EXERCISE

- The Anaerobic-Aerobic Continuum

Weight-training with heavy weights is the classic example of an "Anaerobic" exercise. "An" means "without" and "aerobic" means with "air or oxygen", just like it sounds. When you lift heavy weights with sufficient rest between sets, you usually don't get extraordinarily winded. You get a burn and fatigue in your muscle that brings you to exhaustion in relatively few reps. This process involves energy mechanisms in your muscle that don't require oxygen to burn fuel. This is anaerobic.

"Cardio" is a term of endearment for the type of exercise that stimulates and improves the fitness of your heart. (short for cardiovascular or cardiorespiratory exercise; "cardia" latin for heart). This can also be called "aerobic" exercise which requires oxygen to fuel the muscle movement. Cardio can be done in many forms, but usually involves low resistance exercise utilizing large muscle groups in repetitive movements. The ultimate objective of Cardio is to improve cardiovascular health, efficiency, and performance while burning fat. When you perform cardio, you elevate your heart rate and breathe heavier for a given time with corresponding elevations in energy expenditure.

During this type of training, one utilizes "oxidative" metabolism. That is, oxygen is consumed to produce energy by burning fat stores. This is why Cardio is also called "aerobic" exercise, oxygen is consumed to burn fat while carbon dioxide (CO_2) is produced and expired from the lungs. It is a very energy efficient process and one can go for long periods of time when well trained. Conversely, anaerobic exercise involves a higher intensity that utilizes stored carbohydrate and produces the painful lactic acid in your muscles which comes with "the burn".

Despite what many people think, there is a blurred line between aerobic exercise and anaerobic exercise. Aerobic exercise can become anaerobic if the intensity is elevated to a point where exhaustion is achieved quickly and the lungs can't get enough oxygen to the muscle. For instance, if you run at a steady pace and then sprint to exhaustion you have just converted aerobic to anaerobic exercise. You know this has happened because you become short of breath and must rest from the pain in your muscle. If you aren't bringing in enough oxygen as you get short of breath you can no longer acquire energy from "ox"idative metabolism. Anaerobic activity burns stored carbohydrate (glycogen) and energy stored as creatine -phosphate. (Creatine will be discussed in more detail in "N"utrition)

CARDIO TRAINING ZONES:

If your focus is to improve the health of your heart, then it is important to understand the value of measuring your heart rate. Your heart rate and changes in heart rate from rest to exercise and vice versa is a direct measure of your cardiovascular fitness. As your fitness improves, your heart is able to pump more blood with each beat and thus you have a lower heart rate for the same level of exertion. Thus, an unhealthy person will see greater rises in heart rate with relatively less exertion. There are a few different measurements of heart rate that are important for you to recognize:

- Heart Rate Maximum (HR_{max}) This is the fastest your heart can beat per minute (bpm). To directly measure this you would have to perform a strict stress test with a cardiologist and physiologist. Since this really isn't feasible for most there are a couple of simple ways to measure HR_{max}:

    – The easiest is "Age-Predicted HR_{max}" = [220-your age]

    However, this will often underestimate your true HR_{max}.

    – The "Inbar equation" may be the most accurate prediction based on age is= [$205.8 - 0.685*age$]

- Resting Heart Rate (RHR) Your RHR is how quickly your heart beats at complete rest (i.e. while sleeping or immediately after waking). You can measure it with a heart rate monitor at night or upon waking in the morning. This should be measured on a day when you wake without an alarm and you wake without sitting up first. If you do not have a monitor, measure it for 3 or 4 days and make an average.

– Normal is around 50-60bpm. Very fit athletes may even be in the 40s. By measuring your RHR you can also get a sense of the current condition of your body and training. Rises of 10% or more on waking after a hard training day can indicate that your body is stressed or on the verge of illness or injury. For example if your RHR is normally 60 and you notice that it rises with training to 65 the over the next few mornings you may need to rest or at least take it easier for a day or two until it is back to your average or lower.

- Delta Heart Rate (DHR) The DHR represents the "change" (delta "D" means change) in your HR from sitting to standing or resting to exercising. The DHR is another way to assess your cardiovascular fitness or level of hydration. The simplest way to measure DHR is to take your heart rate after lying down for 2 minutes. Next, stand up and measure your heart rate. If you see a rise of 10-20bpm this is relatively normal (<10 is excellent). If you see a rise of >20bpm this can indicate an overtrained or even dehydrated state. If you get light-headed, hydrate and seek medical attention if it persists.

The DHR can be used from any resting state to any particular exercise. You can standardize this measure any way you would like. For instance, you can measure your heart rate before getting on a treadmill and running at 6mph. Measure your heart rate after 5 minutes of running at that pace. The less your heart rate rises at 5 minutes the

more fit you are. If you come back and do
the same test again and you notice your heart
rate increases more rapidly than previously
(especially >10% more) then you are likely
in an overtrained state and should work
more on your recovery and train lighter until
this improves.

- Heart Rate Recovery (HRR) HRR is a very
  useful measure of cardiovascular fitness.
  It is a measure used reliably by cardiologists
  to determine improvements in heart function
  after heart attacks. It can be used by athletes
  to determine your level of cardiovascular
  fitness and training state (i.e. overtraining).
  HRR is measured by getting your heart rate
  up to 90% of your Heart Rate Maximum on
  a bike or treadmill and then stopping,
  standing still for 2 minutes and measuring
  the rate of decrease in your heart rate. The
  faster your heart rate declines, the more fit
  you are. For instance, if your HRMax
  is 180 and you get your heart rate up to 162
  on a treadmill and step off and measure HR
  after 2 minutes and it is 150. Your HR
  recovered at 6bpm (HRR=6 bpm). If you do
  this challenge again and it decreases from
  162 to 144 your HRR increased to 9bpm and
  you are seeing improvements in your health.
  Again, if you are seeing that HRR is
  decreasing, you may be overtraining or
  becoming ill.

- Target Heart Rate - Your Target Heart Rate
  is your goal for how hard you plan to train
  your heart. The target is a certain percentage
  or range of percentage of your HR_{max}.
  Training at different target heart rates

has different effects on your fitness. Lower target heart rates correspond to fat burning and endurance exercise. Training at a higher target brings in more cardiovascular training and strengthening. Target heart rate zones are as follows:

CALCULATING TRAINING HEART RATES USING THE KARVONEN METHOD

The Karvonnen formula accurately predicts your training zone heart rate by factoring in your resting heart rate. Resting heart rate corresponds well to fitness level, with a lower resting heart rate corresponding to better fitness. If you know your resting heart rate you can more reliably determine the heart rate zone needed to improve your performance and longevity. Again, your resting heart rate can be measured by using *The G.A.I.N. Plan* Monitor or by checking your pulse immediately after waking averaged over 3 days. You can use the online calculators at www.yourgainplan.com or follow the method below.

Step 1: Measure your resting heart rate

Step 2: Calculate your maximum heart rate
220 - your age = HRmax

Step 3: Determine your heart rate reserve (HRr): Subtract your Resting HR from your HRmax.

Step 4: Select your target HR zone (select your goal in the chart above)

	Step 5: Multiply your HRr by your desired intensity range (80% is .8 x HRr) Step 6: Add your RHR to your HRr to determine your target heart rate RATINGS OF PERCEIVED EXERTION Ratings of perceived exertion (RPE) have been made to help you understand what zone you are training in without measuring your heart
Zone 1	50 - 60% of your Maximum Heart Rate. Talk Test: easy to converse or sing. The zone for warm-ups and cool-downs. It is the lowest level of workout that will result in increases in fitness for beginners.
Zone 2 *The "Fat"* *Burning Zone"*	60 - 70% of Maximum Heart Rate you will be in the "Fat Burning Zone." Talk Test: Comfortably able to talk Light jog, steady weight training circuit at low intensity
Zone 3 *The Aerobic* *Zone*	70-80% of Maximum Heart Rate Talk Test: say a short sentence, catch breath, then speak more. Training for endurance performance
Zone 4 *The Anaerobic* *Threshold*	80-90% of Maximum Heart Rate. Talk Test: gasping, difficult to get air. This is where the aerobic-anaerobic continuum breaks down into lactic acid build up and muscles working harder than the heart and lungs can keep up with. Interval training and high intensity CCC puts you in Zone 4. Pace yourself as you can't stay in this zone for long.

| Zone 5 Red Zone | 90-100% of Maximum Heart Rate.

Only for the highest level of athlete in sprint competition. Check with your physician before going to this level of intensity |

rate. However, your perception of exertion is closely tied to your attitude. If you are down in the dumps, lighter exercise is going to seem more difficult than it would if you did the same exercise when well rested and in a positive mental attitude. Your exertion can simply be rated on how when you can breathe and talk during your activity (See Talk Test in above table of HR Zones).

Numerical Rating	Rating in Words	Description
0	Rest	Sitting, lying down
1	Easy	Walking at a slow pace
2	Moderate	Brisk walk, hurrying to get somewhere
3	Hard	Jog and starting to sweat.
4	Very hard	Running
5	Maximal Effort	Running up a hill

HIIT vs LISS

One of the biggest myths that persist in the bodybuilding community is that low intensity aerobic exercise done for long periods of time is the key to burning fat more effectively. This just isn't the case. Some think that there is a target heart rate for fat burning that you shouldn't exceed or you'll just start burning less fat. To a small extent this can be true. As your heart rate increases above 90% of your HR max you lose your breath and fatigue quickly because you exceed the aerobic "oxidative" fat-burning machinery's ability to keep producing energy. But on your way up to that level you have just forced that fat burning machine to work as hard as possible burning *more* fat.

This is where the concept of INTERVAL TRAINING comes in to play. Interval training involves mixing low to moderate intensity exercise with higher intensity exercise into one session. The intervals can be in many different patterns allowing for some variety in your training. Intervals can include alternating 2 minutes of low-moderate intensity with up to 60 seconds of high intensity with many variations in between. The protocols usually involve a 5 minute warm up and 5 minute cool down with 10-20 minutes of intervals. These cardio sessions are typically shorter than your low intensity steady state cardio because they can be exhausting. I love the feeling of accomplishment that I get from intervals.

When done at the highest intensities the intervals are called High Intensity Interval Training or "HIIT". A typical moderate intensity cardio session may include jogging at 6 miles per hour for 45 minutes (4.5miles) at a heart rate of around 130-140. For an active person this is a relatively moderate pace consisting of a 10 minute mile. Now let's say we do a brisk walk at 4 miles per hour and every other minute run all out at 10 miles per hour for 30 seconds. In this training session you may have gone a shorter distance but it is possible that you burned more fat and stimulated more adaptations to exercise than the simple jog.

During the high intensity intervals, it is possible to bring your heart rate up to 80-95% of your maximum. When you go back to walking your heart rate will likely remain elevated throughout a large portion of that walk. In essence your heart rate remains elevated more throughout the exercise despite less distance being covered. Also, those episodes of high intensity have just "SHOCKED" your body into realizing that it needs to grow and adapt to this new stress. This includes boosting secretion of growth hormone from your pituitary and improving the function of the most anabolic hormone: insulin. The metabolic responses after HIIT also contribute to your total caloric burn throughout the day. When the system has been shocked in this fashion, your basal metabolic rate and thus calories burned remains elevated for more than 24 hours!

Low intensity steady state cardio or "LISS" may allow for a greater percentage of energy to be burned as fat rather than total amount of fat burned. LISS may be the ideal form of cardio for you under a number of circumstances. First, it may just be more comfortable and thus more tolerable, albeit slightly boring (get creative). You will not have to work as hard throughout the exercise and you won't have episodes of difficulty catching your breath as can occur with very high intensities.

Bodybuilders prepping for a contest sometimes need to go on a No Carb diet for a brief time. On such depleted diets high intensity cardio can

Invigorate Your LISS

- *Move backwards*
- *Get your arms involved*
- *Dance*
- *Use music*
- *Alternate resistance; mild to moderate*

be too much stress for the hungry bodybuilder trying to make weight. Not to mention some bodybuilders or overweight individuals are quite large and can't handle the impact on their knees or back to do higher intensities of running. HIIT can be done on a bike, elliptical, or rowing machine to avoid the impact on the knees and back, but you may still need to build up slowly. Additionally, intense leg workouts may lead to soreness that limits your ability to do high intensity cardio. In this situation a gradual increase in the grade (degree of incline) on a treadmill or tension on an elliptical can help to bring your heart rate up to moderate levels without adding much impact on your joints.

During sessions of LISS, incorporation of some moderate intensity exercise early in a workout can be beneficial. This uses up your glucose stores (glycogen) earlier in the workout, thus switching you to fat burning for the rest of the workout. In LISS training acts as an adjunct to burning fat. It is not meant to make your heart stronger or improve your performance. In order to boost cardiovascular performance you will need to reach moderate intensity levels >70% of your HR_{max}.

When you think about the amount of calories that you burn in a cardio workout, it really isn't that much. 300 Calories may be just half of one meal. The real benefit of the exercise performed is not gained so much while doing it; it is the responses your body makes to the exercise in the following days that makes a bigger difference. You might say, what about just doing more cardio in a day, i.e. > 1 hour? The problem with extending your cardio training session is that your body may switch on a stress response that elevates cortisol levels which breaks down hard earned muscle. Not to mention the possibility of over-training and stress injuries. Performing HIIT requires shorter training sessions and longer recovery and really shouldn't be done more than 2 to 3 times per week.

The most important aspect of choosing how little cardio you can get away with depends on your goals and the intensity that you apply to the session. If you are looking to get stronger and build speed and power, long runs for 45-60 minutes may actually be detrimental. Shorter 20-30 minute interval programs may provide the endurance building effects, while working the fast twitch muscle fibers that are critical for power. If your goal is fat loss, sessions up to 45 minutes in length may be necessary to burn the fat desired.

The 2 to 3 days a week cardio is great for maintenance and some fat loss especially early in your training program. A 2 to 3 day per week schedule can be plenty for adding a little endurance to strength training routines and for power athletes who want to improve their workout efficiency.

A couple of sessions of cardio can improve your efficiency in taking on the CCC. HIIT is ideal for those who embrace P.A.C.E. With all the varieties of training that you can imagine with HIIT, there are all sorts of impressive feats that you can try to attain. You can try to maintain a desired average heart rate and have challenges with others to do the same. You can try to attain higher peak heart rates or speeds during the high intensity

intervals. It is more fun to compete in intervals
and keep track of progress through distance
covered or peak intensity.

Those who are unaccustomed to cardio of any
type tend to see its benefits relatively quickly.
These results will often start to taper off and
plateau over time. At that point you'll have to
step it up and "SHOCK" the system. This can
be done with either HIIT, increased time on the
machine, and/or increased number of cardio
sessions. Consider the variety and flexibility of
HIIT when LISS would otherwise seem boring
and tedious.

FASTING CARDIO

One of the controversies in nutrition and exercise
is whether to consume carbohydrate prior to fat
burning exercise. Clearly, one should consume
carbohydrates before exercise meant to improve
performance or in competition, but when your
goal is to burn fat instead of performance things
are a bit different. Those who are trying to lose
fat approach their diet with reductions in calories
from carbohydrates or fats. These reductions
can put strain on hard earned muscle and risk
unwanted loss of muscle.

A substantial portion of energy production
during endurance comes from the burning of fat.
When your diet is higher in protein and fat, your
muscle adapts to more effectively utilize fat to
spare muscle glycogen. Furthermore, endurance
training improves your muscle's ability to use
fat for energy sparing muscle glycogen and
protein. If your diet is high in carbohydrate,
the percentage of carbohydrate used during

endurance exercise increases. Carbohydrate oxidation (burning glucose for energy) increases progressively with exercise intensity, whereas the most efficient of fat oxidation is found during exercise at <70% of HR_{max}.

Fat is readily available for energy after a night of sleep as liver glycogen stores are depleted by the overnight fast. Thus, there is less glucose available to burn as fuel and the body muscle go to other sources of fuel like fat or muscle. During endurance exercise fat is released from stores resulting in more fat to be available for working muscles. If a carbohydrate-rich meal is consumed glucose becomes the preferred substrate and fat mobilization enzymes are shut down by the rise in insulin. Insulin commands that the glucose absorbed be converted into stores of fat and glycogen. It can be easily deduced that consuming glucose prior to your exercise intended to burn your fat is counter-productive to your goal. Research supports that fat burning is definitely greater in the fasted state vs. the fed state.

Food fuels the workout instead of stores

That being said, if your endurance training is meant to make you stronger, faster, or more conditioned for distance rather than burning fat, then you should spare your muscle and fat by consuming carbohydrate, at a minimum after your training.

Fasting before endurance training can provide stimulus for improvements in muscle substrate metabolism, and may even be considered as an adjunctive training technique. That is, fasted endurance training improves the contribution of intra-muscular fats used in energy production during endurance training. Fasted training improves the muscle's efficiency to burn fat more than exercise done with similar duration and intensity with adequate carbohydrate intake. Perhaps more importantly for the low-carb dieter, fasted state endurance training prevents the drop in blood glucose seen in exercise after a carbohydrate meal. This avoids the crash that can occur when training after consuming sugars or carbs. Fasted endurance training can add powerful adaptations that can improve endurance performance.

Although some studies show that fasting cardio can lead to greater muscle breakdown for energy the data is not as applicable to *The G.A.I.N. Plan*. Most studies that examined the effects of fasting did not incorporate increased protein intake, anabolic weight training, and anabolic nutritional supplementation. Weight training exercise encourages muscle growth and supplements like creatine monohydrate and HMB have anti-catabolic effects on muscle. Taking a HMB-Leucine supplement prior to your "fasted" cardio in the mornings can help spare muscle breakdown during otherwise fasted cardio.

If you want the fat burning machinery to stay on longer, a low to no carbohydrate diet will maximize mobilization of fat. Based on this science, I recommend performing fasted cardiovascular exercise at moderate intensities before breakfast combined with a low carbohydrate diet when your goal is to lose body fat. When carbohydrates are a part of your *G.A.I.N. Plan* the timing of their consumption is maximized to spare muscle and lose fat. For instance, consuming carbs after your weight training session is recommended. Avoiding situations where your carbohydrate consumed is most likely to be stored as fat is the key. Therefore consumption of carbohydrates before periods of relative inactivity such as at rest or sleeping is avoided. I will go over nutrient timing in a little more detail in the "N"utrition section.

STRETCHING

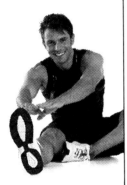

Flexibility is very important in any exercise routine. Stretching exercises are very important for keeping joints supple, maintaining range of motion, and recovery from muscle soreness. As a gymnast and martial artist (Tae Kwon Do), I have always appreciated how stretching helped me to loosen up and stay limber.

Science has shown that this is the wrong approach. Researchers have found that static stretching where you hold a stretch for 10-30 seconds is an inadequate way to warm up leading to decreased performance and potential injury to the muscles stretched. Rather, it is important to do an active warm-up getting blood flowing to the muscles and joints. Statically holding a stretch can actually limit blood flow to a body part. Thus it is suggested that before going for a vigorous run, do some light jogging for a few minutes as opposed to just sitting and stretching your hamstrings. Before you bench press, do some pushups. That being said, there is a role for stretching and flexibility exercises after your training or at another time in the day. *It is important to recognize that static stretching before high intensity or impact exercise is not recommended.*

Types of Stretching:

a. STATIC STRETCHING

This is where you stretch a particular muscle
for a hold of 15 to 30 seconds without
bouncing or moving. It should produce a
mild, painless pulling sensation in the muscle
and not hurt your joints

b. DYNAMIC STRETCHING

Stretching style where you swing your legs
or arms through a stretched position at your
limits of range of motion. Speed can be
gradually increased.

c. BALLISTIC STRETCHING

This stretching forces a body part to go
beyond its normal range of motion by
bouncing in to a stretched position. It triggers
the muscle's stretch reflex (and thus muscle
relaxation), but can make you more
susceptible to injury if done by the
inexperienced.

d. PASSIVE STRETCHING

This is basically static stretching with a partner
who helps hold you in a stretched position.
They can add a little extra stretch or get you
into a position you might not be able to on
your own.

e. ACTIVE ISOLATED STRETCHING

This involves holding a limb in a position
without assistance of another limb or partner.
For instance, holding your leg up in the air
without using your hands or a support.

f. ISOMETRIC STRETCHING

Similar to static stretching, but during this stretch you contract the stretched muscle to resist the stretching movement.

g. PROPRIOCEPTIVE NEUROMUSCULAR FACILITATION

This is a combination of static, passive, and isometric stretching. First, you stretch in a static position. Then you perform an isometric contraction resisted by your partner for ~10 seconds. After the contraction your partner passively stretches you past your last static position. This is a very advanced form of stretching.

Individual Stretching Routine:

a. Warm-up Jumping Jacks or Jog in Place for 1 minute

b. Standing Quad Stretch 15 sec each leg x 3

c. Achilles Stretch each leg 15 sec x 3

d. Hamstring Stretches: hold 30 seconds x 3

e. Straddle Stretch: hold 15 sec x3 Left, Middle, and Right alternating

f. Arch Ups to Crunch 15 sec in each position x 3

g. Overhead Lat Stretch each arm 15 sec x3

h. Behind the Back Chest Stretch hold 30 sec

i. Behind the Head Triceps Stretch 15 sec x 3

j. Cross arm Rear Deltoid Stretch 15 sec x

2. A: Attitude

The Power of Attitude

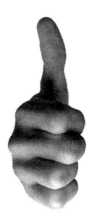

My coach always told me that gymnastics was 90% mental and 20% physical. That's right, you must give 110%.

Of all the pillars of *The G.A.I.N.Plan*, attitude is inherently pervasive in the plan, but probably the hardest to evaluate and change. Your attitude affects not only you, but the world around you. Your attitude can affect your performance in the gym and your actions in the gym can affect your attitude. Your attitude affects how you look at food and whether you make healthy choices or not. When your attitude is trending more negative than yesterday, you tend to perceive the same exertion as more laboring than yesterday. Negative attitude causes you to eat more inappropriate foods and you create bad habits.

How do we end up with a negative attitude? When you bite off more than you can chew, your mind is taxed and your stress levels rise. If you do too much too soon and too often you will crush your positivity in a crippling way. Stress, anxiety, and depressed mood lead to an inability to move forward and become better than yesterday's self. Your attitude and thus your mind need active rest and recovery just like your body. Without proper recovery, it is hard to refresh your attitude and turn it around. Inadequate sleep, stress management, or nutrition all lead to attitude deterioration. I want to help you to recognize your attitude and its effects on your body and mind. Through proactive attitude adjustment, we can make "today's self" better than yesterday's.

Your Attitude Affects Your World

Your attitude is perceived by others and they respond accordingly. If you are being positive and upbeat, those around you will often respond favorably. Ever hear that a smile is contagious? Just try smiling at a stranger when you are walking down the street. Have you ever bought a big bouquet of flowers? Have you appreciated the smiles people project while you are carrying them? Try it sometime and pay attention to those around you.

Of course the opposite is also true, negative attitudes are contagious. Negative attitudes are projected through words, actions, and facial expressions and can be projected on others like a mirror. Have you ever worked in an environment where your boss is unhappy and bitter? The office shares that negative mentality and morale tends to be quite low. Similarly, negative attitudes tend to attract negative people. Negativistic thinking leads you to attract others who wish to wallow in their troubles with you. This will only put you into a cycle of negative thinking that becomes hard to break.

If you think negatively, you will often seek confirmation that your situation is bleak. I often notice this with friends going through romantic relationship troubles? They almost always start out with a feeling that their partner could "be the one" and that they are "perfect." However, as the relationship becomes more familiar and soured, your friend may start to mention how certain things piss them off. The more you agree with them, affirming the negative, the more it affirms their negative feelings for their partner.

This is a cycle that is hard to break unless you recognize it and actively change the direction of the conversation. You could be the friend who reminds them of why they fell in love in the first place and renew their positive attitudes toward each other.

I was trapped in a similar cycle during my residency training. Residency is a challenging time of learning, personal criticism, long hours, humbling stress, and physical demands. It is very easy to wallow in a negative sense of self when you are being bossed around by others not much older and sometimes less intelligent. It is also easy to forget that your training program is world renowned and very difficult to gain acceptance into. At times, I became so negative that I just wanted to pack my bags and head back to Chicago. Our chairman was so controlling at times that the resident morale hit many low points where all the residents wanted to leave. However, every year of my training there was a time where my attitude was lifted and my desire to train harder was renewed. That time of year was the week of residency interviews.

During resident interviews, we would meet over a hundred different medical students who were putting their best foot forward to get in the door with energy and enthusiasm. Likewise, we as a residency program were trying to sell the idea that we had the best program in the country and only the best students would be accepted. I always wanted to make it sound like we were being trained better than anyone else and that it was a unique privilege to be a part of the program. The medical students would try to convince us that they felt the same about our program and that they would work harder than the next because it was just in their nature. Listening to lectures given by our chairman and personally describing the success of the program to others made it impossible to leave the interviews without a sense of pride and accomplishment. Even when I was over-stressed, putting on that face of pride helped adjust my attitude to the positive. If I could just sell my program every day, I would love my program every day. So, why not sell it every day?

Perhaps more damaging is that if you expect negative results, you are less likely to take risks and try new things. Negative thinking results in fear of failure and fear of the unknown. Positive thinking helps you move past fear trying things that others may believe "can't be done". My coach at Michigan State, Rick Atkinson, an intense and jovial fellow, always knew that I embraced this concept. He would use "reverse psychology" on me. In other words, he would tell me something negative knowing that I would turn into a positive challenge. He would say things like, "a perfectly level inverted iron cross is impossible on the rings" or "the Victorian cross is physically impossible". He did this, jokingly, knowing that I would find these statements motivating. I wanted to prove him wrong! Of course, by the end of that season I performed a perfectly level inverted cross and competed with the Victorian cross for the first time in modern NCAA history. It took a lot of hard work and ignoring my few negative teammates who thought it was crazy for me to spend as much time as I did on doing these things. I kept a positive attitude and often had daydreams about performing those skills. I visualized myself doing those skills with perfection even though I had never seen them done before. I truly believe that a person's thinking determines their reality.

Anyone who accomplishes anything, whether it is making a million dollars or finishing a marathon, accomplishes it by believing in themselves and taking action. Positive thinkers have a leg up because they believe the object of their desire is attainable and they take action, no matter how little that initial action. Negative thinkers are often defeated before they even start because of paralyzing fear and lack of self-esteem. Only belief in success and ultimately reward will motivate one to act on goals and desires.

See Things In a Different Light

Positive thinking puts your situation in a different light, even though it doesn't really change your situation. We all need rose colored glasses. Positivity makes you realize that your situation CAN change and WILL change with hard work. Hard work seems easier as you know that it will lead you closer to your goals no matter how much pain it inflicts.
For instance, getting upset about your soreness after a workout will only distract you from finding adjustments to move forward. Getting upset with an injury is just as unproductive. If you are injured look at the positives and grow from the experience.

When I started my bodybuilding career, I was overly excited and motivated to succeed. In my first year I achieved my goal of competing on a national stage and obtaining a sponsorship with *Muscletech*. However, shortly after my success,

I had the accident where I tore my bicep tendon. Initially I was upset and discouraged. These feelings of defeat were quickly replaced by a new positive outlook.

My upper body was very well developed from competing in gymnastics, especially on the rings. However, my lower body was far behind and held me back from placing higher in bodybuilding. I never trained legs like a bodybuilder when I was a gymnast because they would weigh me down on the rings. In fact, I spent many hours in the off season working on bringing my leg size down with endurance running while building my upper body on the rings.

My bicep injury resulted in new motivation. First, it forced me to focus on building my lower body. For the first time, I would learn to really train my legs like a bodybuilder with high volume and intensity. Second, it made me set a goal to be back on stage like nothing happened within 6 months after the injury. Ultimately I came back to compete in exactly 6 months without judges knowing that I tore my bicep. In fact, I placed higher in the national level show than I did the year before.

So when something seems like a negative, especially an injury, turn it around and make it into a life lesson. In a sense, positive mental attitude changes your reality by allowing you to act in an entirely different way and leads to entirely different results.

Just remember that with every situation whether it is positive or negative will give you a chance to respond. If you respond negatively, you can spiral into a cycle of despair. If you respond in the positive you will grow and be stronger. Try this exercise in self-motivation.

1.   Write down how something negative in your life has led to something positive:

_____

_____

2.   Write down something negative going on in your life right now that you can change for the better:

_____

_____

Trauma and Success

My favorite quotes: "*Pain is weakness leaving the body.*" "*Whatever doesn't kill you only makes you stronger.*" "*Pain is temporary, Pride is forever.*"

Sometimes motivational speakers and positive thinkers may seem flighty and even cheesy. I admit it is difficult to discuss PMA without feeling like I am a happy-go-lucky motivator. That being said it is important to realize that being a positive person doesn't mean that I expect life to be perfect. In fact, I expect life to be difficult and challenging. I embrace challenges and setbacks as these are where I have grown the most in my life.

When I left the Air Force Academy, I thought my life was in a downward spiral, but I fought for a scholarship and worked hard in college to meet my goals. I learned to make difficult decisions in my own best interest. I learned to sell my best qualities to those who wanted to buy them. I've felt a great sense of accomplishment having jumped the hurdle of what I once thought was a failure.

I came back from being wait-listed to medical school to graduate at the top of my class proving to the admissions committee that they were wrong about me (they should've taken me first!). I didn't have a doctor in the family to "talk" to someone at the school. I didn't have the money to pay for medical school or parents who could afford to help. If everything in life had gone "perfectly" and everything was handed to me on a platter, I wouldn't have such a great sense of personal accomplishment or the tools to pass on to you.

In order for you to adapt and improve your performance at any endeavor, you must embrace that your journey won't always be a perfect. Perfectionism is a valuable virtue and an annoyance. As great as it feels to do things without making mistakes, those mistakes are valuable lessons waiting to be learned.

"No one cares how hard you fell, but they can be impressed by how quickly you get up."

Some think that when they are in intense training they should protect themselves from extraneous pressures in order to focus on the task at hand. Athletes or their coaches and parents may try to put them in a "bubble", so to speak, protecting them from the pressures of the outside world. Unfortunately, this is counterproductive leading to a lack of resources for negotiating future stressors. Resilience, mental toughness, and the "growth mind-set" are all concepts that have been researched and are considered to be psychological characteristics of developing excellence.

Many high level successful athletes can recall 'influential low points' in their careers the details of which are often quite vivid. This could be an injury that changed focus, a life stressor such as death of a family member, or an extended period away from the gym that led to rejuvenation of the competitive spirit. Those who have resilience will grow from adversity and be more prepared when adversity rears its head again. Just as shocking your body makes your muscles grow, stressful events build resiliency. Just as we discussed with your muscles, you need to actively recover from those stressful events. I will describe ways to recover in the sections to come.

Learning from adversity leads to self-discipline and self-control. These two virtues are thought to play a causative role in achievement. In fact, there is scientific evidence that characteristics of self-discipline and self-control are strong predictors of academic achievement, weight control, and long-term desired behaviors. Research predicts that intermittent exposure to life stressors followed by periods of adaptation and adjustment before new challenges fosters a new set of skills and attitudes that strengthen the individual for future experiences. Research also shows that learning from these experiences leads to a different hormonal response to stress characterized by solution-focused perceptions. Again, proof that our minds control our physiology.

Coaches often employ stressors in training to improve the ability to deal with adversity in competition. My gymnastics coach at Iowa State loved to use such tactics. For instance, I might have been practicing my pommel horse routine and out of nowhere a foam block from the pit gets thrown into my legs. This would push me off balance and require adjustments that I normally wouldn't have to make during the routine. This takes the mind out of autopilot and makes you an active participant in the performance. Other sports such as football incorporate similar techniques such as training in an indoor field with simulated noise to mimic the deafening audience of a game in a dome, training in the rain, altitude training, or training at night.

This is where *The G.A.I.N. Plan* fits in. In the plan I recommend reaching milestones in a linear fashion KNOWING that failure might occur. We need to try and anticipate obstacles to progress and have action plans in place. *The G.A.I.N. Plan* was developed to provide you with tools to help you prepare and overcome obstacles to become resilient and successful. Negotiating plateaus in a timely fashion is critical to continued success. Shocking the system teaches you about how your body and mind react to such stress helping you grow from the experience. As an example, putting myself into the 90% heart rate max training zone, I learn to control my breathing and realize that I'm not going to pass out at this level. I learn that I can recover and I will be able to reach this level in competition without catastrophic failure. Put this "can do" mindset to work for you in your training.

Accepting Change

To keep moving toward your goals you need to accept change. If you are complacent and resistant to change you will not grow in body or mind. Just as your body must experience graded exercise, so must your dreams. Change comes with challenges and stress.

Think of how a 3 year old sees the world. Everything they do is new and they often don't know what to fear. They get to experience something new every day. They are always smarter than yesterday's self. They don't judge themselves with failure and they try things over and over, especially if they get a desired result. We must find and embrace our "inner 3 year old" and grow in mind, body, and spirit every day. Every moment has potential to be a gift or a lesson.

So am I preaching to the choir? You are already motivated to read this, so what do we need to teach you? When you think about this moment, you can get a great sense of pride knowing that you are already moving in the right direction. However, there will be times when life challenges you and it can be very easy to get frustrated and discouraged. You will need a bag of tricks to keep you from the downward spiral of despair. It may be very difficult during those times to sit and open a self-help book.

The G.A.I.N. Plan will be an easy access reference to techniques which can bring you back on track in "G.A.I.N."ing self-confidence and self-motivation. If the book isn't enough, look to yourgainplan.com for message boards filled with fellow positive thinkers to boost your goals.

When in a frustrating situation ask yourself:

1. Is there a gift in this situation?
2. Is there anything to learn from the situation?
3. Is there any way to change things for the better?

Take Action:

If you learn that something needs to change, start changing it. Don't expect all the change to occur all at once. Do it with one piece at a time (just like eating an elephant). In deciding whether to take action you may realize that there is nothing you can do to change things. In this case, you have to let the situation roll off your back like water on a duck. Making big stinks about things that you cannot change is like taking 5 steps forward and 6 steps back; it is a lot of wasted time and energy. One of the toughest lessons in life is learning to understand when a situation isn't within your control and learning to accept the things we cannot change.

PMA and CBT

Cognitive behavioral therapy (CBT) is a technique utilized by psychiatrists and psychologists to achieve 2 goals:

1. Help you feel better in the here and now— BUILD PMA
2. Help you develop a realistic personal value system with utilities to improve mood and deal with conflict.

Your thoughts and attitudes, not external events, create your feelings about the world around you. CBT is designed to help you recognize when you need to change the way you are thinking to improve your feelings and behavior. Depressive or anxious feelings are often a result of pessimistic and self-critical thoughts that need to be changed to positive, realistic, and productive thoughts. CBT is excellent for addressing mood problems and feelings of inferiority. It is not meant to provide intellectual rationalizations for your feelings. CBT is meant to bring you into feelings of well-being.

Although some negative thoughts are real and deserve acknowledgement (i.e. death of a loved one), other thoughts can lead us to be conned into misery and self-doubt. For instance, you may "con" yourself into believing that your father died from lung cancer because you didn't force him to quit smoking when you were younger. These feelings of inadequacy or personal blame are only self-defeating and can't fix the problem. Through CBT, you can learn to overcome these obstacles to positive thinking. The principles of this technique are quite simple, but the actual procedures and action plans to improve your way of thinking can be quite involved and require a great deal of effort. Often, when your negativism feels deeply engrained, one might need to seek professional help from a psychologist or psychiatrist. There are biological reasons for negative thinking that can benefit from treatment with medication. Unfortunately, this discussion goes beyond the scope of this book.

I certainly don't expect feelings of happiness all the time. I don't expect you to be an emotional robot.

It is impossible to be in control of your feelings 24/7. Having appropriately negative thoughts as in times of injury or uncontrolled adversity is a part of being human. Adversity brings us closer and allows us to share feelings. These experiences are an opportunity for personal growth, creativity, and intimacy.

Cognitive Distortions and CBT

The first aspect of CBT is identifying the cognitive distortions that lead to negative and destructive thinking. These distortions need to be identified before you can see the truth in how you are feeling. Dr. David Burns described these 10 forms of "Twisted Thinking" in his book, *The Feeling Good Handbook*. Read through these distortions and try to be critical of yourself and your own tendency to employ these distortions:

1.   ALL OR NOTHING THINKING

    a. This is when perfectionism can be a hindrance. If you plan to be perfect and you fall just short of achieving perfection an "All or Nothing" distortion would be seeing your effort as a complete failure with no benefit to you or others.

    b. An example might be if you break down and have a cheat meal. "An All or Nothing" distortion would make you binge for the next 3 days because you feel that you completely ruined the diet from one cheat meal. When in reality, one cheat meal would be easy to recover from, whereas the binging, not so much.

2.   OVERGENERALIZATION

   a.   The "always happens to me" or "I never have any success" mentality.

   b.   This is like taking 2nd place at a national show. You had to be successful to get there. Just because you didn't win doesn't mean you will never win, you are only 1 place away from winning. Keep going!

3.   MENTAL FILTER

   a.   Your mental filter only allows the negative to come through.

   b.   For instance, you get an evaluation at work with many positive comments, but you dwell on the one negative comment.

4.   DISCOUNTING THE POSITIVE

   a.   Rejecting a positive critique or event as "must've been a fluke" or "that doesn't count"

   b.   This is purely negativistic thinking. Embrace the positive in everything!

5.   JUMPING TO CONCLUSIONS

   a.   Mind Reading: without asking, just assuming that someone is thinking negatively about you.
      You can't read minds!

   b.   Fortune-telling: you determine that no matter what you do, your action will have a bad outcome
      You can't see the future!

6. MAGNIFICATION

   a. Exaggerating the importance of
      a particular problem or problems, while
      minimizing the positive.

   b. If you magnify the problem, it will block
      your vision of the solution.

7. EMOTIONAL REASONING

   a. Apply your negative emotions to
      a conclusion.

   b. I'm afraid to ride an elevator, thus
      elevators must be dangerous.

8. "SHOULD STATEMENTS"

   a. Saying, "I should do something" is
      a way of making you feel guilt and
      frustration for not doing it. "Shoulds" and
      "Musts" give you a resentful feeling and a
      desire to be rebellious.

   b. Should statements often come with "but".
      "I should go to the gym, but I think I'll
      take a nap instead." You will feel guilty for
      taking the nap.

9. LABELING

   a. Label yourself a "fool" or a "loser" for one
      mistake or failure.

   b. Very similar to overgeneralization and All-
      or-Nothing Thinking.

10. PERSONALIZATION AND BLAME

   a. Holding yourself personally responsible
      for a negative event that was out of
      your control.

    b. Your father dies of lung cancer. You blame it on being a bad daughter because you didn't force him to quit smoking.

Your thoughts, not external events in your life, determine your mood. Negative thoughts lead to negative feelings and physical stress. Negative thoughts that make you anxious or depressed are often of the distorted type listed above. Recognizing these truths is the first step in breaking out of a bad mood.

Once you have recognized that you are in a negative mood, try writing down what is upsetting you. Writing down your thoughts is the only way to capture them in a way that you can take a step back and see them for their real substance. When you feel down or upset over something write down what is upsetting you. Analyze your thought to see if any of the thought distortions can be applied. If so, ask yourself why you are applying that distortion. Who are you trying to please other than yourself? What would give you satisfaction in this situation? Just writing these things down can be eye-opening and therapeutic.

When looking at your mood from a practical view point, it may be difficult to know if you should accept your feelings for what they are, express your feelings to others, or change your feelings. Dr. Burns suggests you ask yourself these questions:

1. ***How long have I been feeling this way?***

    a. Are you feeling bad about something from the past that can't be changed? What is the point of feeling bad for so long? Why let your thoughts put your happiness in jail for 10 years, you must move on.

2. **Am I doing something constructive about the problem?**

   a. Are you avoiding your problems or hopeless about changing your life?

3. **Are my thoughts and feelings realistic?**

   a. Identify distortions in your negative thoughts.

4. **Will it help or hurt to express my feelings?**

   a. T.H.I.N.K. before you speak: Is what you are going to share *True*, *Helpful*, *Inspiring*, *Necessary*, and *Kind*?

5. **Am I making myself unhappy about something outside my control?**

   a. Learn to accept what you can't change. You can't change the past!

6. **Am I avoiding a problem or denying that something is upsetting?**

7. **Are my expectations of the world realistic?**

   a. Trains aren't always on time, some will be late.

8. **Are my expectations of myself realistic?**

   a. Perfectionism often complicates this question.

9. *Am I feeling helpless?*

a. Always a distorted assessment of your future

10. *Am I experiencing a loss of self-esteem?*

Again, take the time to write the answers to these questions down when you are feeling depressed or anxious. It can be quite revealing about how your brain works. It is always easier to challenge your thoughts when they are written down. Otherwise it is quite easy to move from one thought to another losing sight of the true problem. When you find that you have significant distortions in your thoughts, spend time being more rational about them and try to see the positive aspects of your situation. Use a negative experience as a way to grow and benefit, instead of defeating yourself.

Here are some cognitive therapy tools that Dr. Burns recommends to keep in your armamentarium. Study these methods and use them to overcome your negative thoughts and feelings.

1. *IDENTIFY YOUR DISTORTIONS.*

Just the act of identifying your distortions can be therapeutic.

2. *EXAMINE THE EVIDENCE.*

Are things really as bad as you think? Are you really a loser in the grand scheme of things? Is everyone around your really better looking?

3. **THE DOUBLE-STANDARD MODEL:**

   If a friend shared his negative thoughts, would I be supportive or put him down? Why would you put yourself down? Treat yourself as well as you would treat your friends.

4. **THE EXPERIMENTAL TECHNIQUE:**

   Is there an experiment you could do to test your negative thought? i.e. Do people really not like you? Send out invitations to a dinner outing and see how many people accept your invitation.

5. **THINKING IN SHADES OF GRAY.**

   Avoid all or nothing, black and white thinking.

6. **THE SURVEY METHOD.**

   Ask would other people agree that this thought is valid?

7. **DEFINE TERMS YOU ARE USING IN YOUR THOUGHTS.**

   Avoid generalities and define what you are labeling yourself. What is a loser? What is a fool? Do you really fit that definition?

8. **THE SEMANTIC METHOD:**

   Avoiding "should statements". Instead of saying, "I should go on a diet" say, "It would be to my advantage to go on a diet"

9. **RE-ATTRIBUTION.**

   Find ways to adjust thoughts of self-blame to rational thoughts of what other factors contributed to the problem.

10. ***COST-BENEFIT ANALYSIS.***

> This is essentially a pros and cons list of why you are having a particular thought. Make 2 columns: "Advantages of Believing This" and "Disadvantages of Believing This"

This process really can be the most challenging aspect of *The G.A.I.N. Plan*. It is mentally and emotionally demanding. If you spend the time to go through this and you aren't having any revelations, you may want to try going through this with a mental health professional. Just writing this section has helped me to identify some cognitive distortions leading to anxiety that I just don't need to be having! Perhaps you will have the same experience?

Fatigue and Perceived Exertion

Sometimes you just feel down in the dumps and can't even imagine going to the gym or cooking healthy food. These feelings of fatigue, depression, and negativism can be a result of mental exhaustion or physical exhaustion. When you are over-stressed by work, family, or emotions you get a feeling of fatigue. When you have over-trained in the gym you get feelings of fatigue and depressed mood. Recognizing your mood and how it affects your performance can be critical to avoiding over-training and associated injuries. (See Integrated Medicine)

Your muscle's ability to perform can be subject to two forms of fatigue:

Peripheral Fatigue: Loss of energy substrates, over exertion

Central Fatigue: Reduced output from the brain

Your level of exercise intensity depends on recruitment of more muscle fibers to keep up with increasing demand. To do this more nerves need to fire bringing in more involvement of the central nervous system. The increases in nerve recruitment eventually increase the sense of "perceived exertion". In other words you FEEL like you are working harder. That perception involves your mind which will also fatigue as does the output from your nervous system and the fuel in your muscles.

Feelings of motivation or self-efficacy can affect your perception of exertion. Additionally, distractions or emotional stressors can affect your processing of that exertion. For instance, when exercise performance is compared between a happy vs. a sad state in the same individual, the sad individual fatigues faster and recruits less muscle fibers during the activity. Research has attributed multiple physiologic factors that the body sends to the brain affecting perception of fatigue or exertion. This includes lactic acid, free-radicals, increased temperature, and dehydration.

By combining nutritional techniques and "brain training" perceptions of fatigue can be minimized to enhance performance and tolerance to exercise. For instance, multiple studies have shown how supplements like creatine monohydrate improve muscle performance by limiting peripheral fatigue. Additionally, adequate hydration and restoration of muscle glycogen (glucose stores) help to limit perceived exertion. I recommend the use of ratings of perceived exertion (RPEs) to assess your attitude when implementing *The G.A.I.N. Plan.*

Try this test to see if you are experiencing central and peripheral fatigue.

The Standardized Exercise Test:

1. Step on a treadmill and walk at 3mph for 2 minutes. Check your heart rate.

2. Increase the speed to a run that you find difficult. (i.e. 8 mph)

3. Run for 3 minutes.

4. Go back to 3 mph and immediately check your heart rate and record your level of perceived exertion based on a scale from 0 to 100. (0= resting, no exertion, 100= need to stop you're going to pass out).

5. After a month of training go back and repeat the above test at the same speeds and time. Record your heart rate and perceived exertion again.

6. If your perceived exertion is that of more work and your heart rate is the same or lower, chances are that you are experiencing more "central fatigue". If your perceived exertion is the same or higher and your heart rate is also higher you are probably experiencing a combination of central and peripheral fatigue. If you are having significant fatigue, evaluate your life-stressors and perform some active recovery through rest/sleep, meditation, stress management, and diet adjustment.

You can do a similar test using a weight lifting exercise. For instance, you can pick a weight on bench press that you can grunt out 10 reps with.

After a few weeks of training the bench press or chest exercises, you can come back to that same weight and see if you find that your perceived exertion is less or if you can crank out a few more reps. If you are improving, then that is great! If your feelings of perceived exertion are worse or you are unable to complete the 10 reps, then you are likely fatigued centrally or peripherally. You need a break. This would include relative rest from chest training, stress relieving techniques, and possibly medical management.

P.A.C.E. and The Selfie!

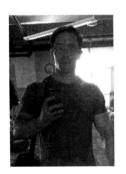

Social media has become a very popular way to find personal motivation. Instagram, Facebook, and Twitter (and others) are great ways to connect to people and share your progress and accomplishments with the world. The "selfie", a picture or video of yourself that you share on social media, has become a way to stay motivated and share your progress with the world. When you post your progress your friends, and even strangers, give you motivational congratulatory words or "likes" that keep you moving forward. Many physique athletes/bodybuilders are exhibitionists to begin with, thus the reason they like to step on stage. These are the folks who really like to take pictures in the bathroom mirror showing the world their abs. For some this is how they use performance as a competitive event (P.A.C.E.). By performing in the world of social media they can stay motivated.

I enjoy using social media to show my creativity and continued athletic achievement. This motivates me to do more. One way that I do this is by posting pictures or videos of my variations on the core CCC exercises. I'll post a variation of chin-ups in a lever position on Instagram or my blog at yourgainplan.com. When I am filming these exercises I use especially good technique and push myself to complete more reps than I typically would without being filmed. It's not that I slack when I am training without the camera, I just find the camera motivating. Knowing that the world can see my workouts makes me try to impress the world. I enjoy being a performer!

Harnessing the performer in you will increase your performance. Whether through the social media stage, entering a contest or just training with your partner harnessing your competitive spirit is a great way to break through plateaus in your training. Try making videos of your training and watch videos of others training. This can be very educational. You will realize when your form sucks or maybe even impress yourself with how good you look. Sharing the video with others can elicit critiques and motivational comments. There are plenty of experienced athletes out there that love to give free advice on social media. It may not always be the best advice, but at least it gives you something to look up in *The G.A.I.N. Plan*.

You can follow me at:

Instagram: instagram.com/victorprisk
Facebook: facebook.com/victor.prisk
Twitter: twitter.com/victorprisk
Blog: yourgainplan.com

PMA and The 3 Goals:

MAINTAINING.

If you are interested in maintaining your current level of fitness, you are likely in a positive place as you have accomplished your goal. However, as we mentioned before, all plateaus erode over time. If you feel good at this plateau and lose motivation to stay there, you will lose what you have GAINED.

Remaining motivated may be a little harder at this level. As I see it, when I've achieved a physique that I like, I end up having less motivation to make changes to my routine. However, you can't forget the basic principles we have outlined earlier. Particularly, you must continue to shock the system with changes in intensity and variety of exercises. This variety not only stimulates maintenance of muscle mass and keeps fat at bay, but it refreshes your mind and keeps you in a positive place.

Intense exercise produces metabolic byproducts and signaling molecules like BDNF that stimulate positive responses in the brain. Once you have reached your goal using techniques like HIIT, you can't become complacent and start doing just LISS. Once you reach a strength goal you will lose it if you don't keep hitting the weights just as hard. Find motivation in maintaining your goal knowing that if you don't use it, you'll lose it.

MUSCLE BUILDING.

Building muscle or improving performance takes a special mentality. You have to have a desire to push your body to new limits. You need to recognize that post-workout soreness isn't the end of the world. I see a number of athletes try to push through muscle soreness and over-training to the point of injury. This leads to significant discouragement. All the PMA in the world with blind ambition leads to injuries like the one I sustained on Muscle Beach.

The muscle builder needs to focus on relative rest and recovery of muscle groups even when they think they are falling behind in their training. The bodybuilder preparing for a show may think they need to hit the gym twice per day because they feel like they're a month behind. This is distorted thinking that leads to overtraining. These are the ones who need to follow *The G.A.I.N. Plan* or get a coach to keep them on track.

The muscle building mentality of "no pain, no gain" requires proper interpretation. This is a very motivating phrase that gets you to lift heavier in the gym. We will discuss how to recognize good vs. bad pain in the Integrated Medicine section. Briefly, the burning pain that you get in your muscles with fatigue and the pain you get the next day (DOMS) are pains that are encouraged to build muscle. They tell you that your workouts are intense enough to evoke adaptations. However, if you don't let those adaptations occur with relative rest you will injure the muscle and end up in a depressed mood related to Over-training Syndrome (OTS; see Integrated Medicine).

FAT BURNING MENTALITY.

Burning fat often requires a small component of caloric restriction. This comes in the form of less food and/or more exercise. Unfortunately, this leads to a little bit of hunger (minimized with the 5MAD *G.A.I.N. Diet*) and a desire to eat poorly. This desire is greatest when first embarking on your goal to burn fat.

The initial discomfort in starting a fat burning program may come from overcoming your addiction to wheat and/or sugar. The cravings for breads and sweets can be overwhelming to some. This can take mindfulness/meditation and even counseling to overcome. Some find it easier to just withdrawal unhealthy foods cold-turkey while others need a gradual wean. I know that I have to do it cold turkey because if I get a taste of bread after removing it for a week it starts to taste like cake, thus becoming more enticing.

The most difficult challenge for the "fat burner" is when the scale stops dropping. Sometimes the scale can fool you if you start gaining muscle. As you burn fat, if you are training hard you may be maintaining more muscle.Muscle weighs more than fat for the same volume; muscle is more dense. In this case it would be better to be measuring your body-fat percentage. Otherwise, a plateau on the scale may mean a lack of variety or intensity in your training or diet. Use this as a motivation to make changes rather than making it into a disappointment. Continue to objectively grade your progress and adjust accordingly.

3. I: Integrated Medicine

The French philosopher Voltaire stated that *"The art of medicine consists of amusing the patient while nature cures the disease."*

The amazing thing about the human body is that it has an incredible ability to regenerate and heal itself. If your body and mind are healthy from exercise, proper diet, and stress control it is really hard to debilitate. Your health is integrated throughout *The G.A.I.N. Plan.* I want you to reach your goals without compromising your health, well-being, and longevity.

We know that daily exercise will help your brain health, heart health, and bone health. We know that stress control will help boost your immune system and brain function. We know that a proper diet will prevent obesity, metabolic syndrome, and a multitude of other medical problems. Even if your goal is to gain weight, every recommendation made throughout this book has your health in mind.

One of the more unique aspects that The G.A.I.N. Plan brings to its participants is the integration of evidence based medical principles. Clearly, this isn't offered by many other programs that are based on expert opinion. As you might have already noticed, *The G.A.I.N. Plan* provides you with a solid scientific foundation for its principles and concepts.

When I prepared for bodybuilding shows, I had a distinct advantage over my gymnastics preparation as I was already a practicing physician. By knowing how changes in diet and training result in changes in human physiology and recovery, I had greater ability to critically analyze my progress. It also gave me a sense of when injury was brewing and how to avert impending disaster.

However, when I first started bodybuilding my focus to succeed led to an overly enthusiastic drive or blind ambition. I ignored my attitude changes, painful tendons, and nutritional balance. That lack of attention to detail led to my bicep rupture that I described in the Birth of G.A.I.N. The objective of The G.A.I.N. Plan is to provide you with the tools to avoid the same injuries I experienced and see in my office every day.

Understanding and appreciating your general health from a medical perspective is critical to your longevity in sport and life. Now, I'm not implying that you need to go through medical school, I couldn't even afford it nowadays, but some basic medical knowledge can go a long way. For instance, you may lack appreciation for when pain is potentially injurious. Are you just sore or do you have an evolving injury? Does everyday stress increase your risk of injury? Do your pre-existing conditions prevent you from exercising at all? What measurements indicate better heart health? With some very basic understanding and monitoring of the benefits and even the risks of diet, exercise, and behavioral change you can direct you down the path of success.

Practicing Medicine

The "practice" of medicine fits in well with the pillars of *The G.A.I.N. Plan* as it to puts plenty of practice into your plan. The concept of "practicing" medicine means that we are always trying to improve our abilities, techniques, and science. Doctors are expected to periodically "grade" themselves and participate in what is called Continuing Medical Education (CME). Conscientious physicians even grade their day to day outcomes either by keeping detailed records or by participating in research studies.

Dr. Bill Hamilton: "*Nothing spoils good results like having a fellow look them up.*"

Without constant self-evaluation, it is very difficult to keep an objective view of your outcomes in medical practice. Most physicians, especially surgeons like me, believe that they perform better than they really do. When results of our procedures are objectively reviewed we often discover room for improvement. Innovators of health care recognize the need for improvement making adjustments based on their objective data. When we practice based on solid scientific evidence, we are practicing "evidence based medicine".

Some evidence is stronger than others. High level studies involve removal of bias by blinding the researcher and the subject of treatments used. Studies like the "double blind" "randomized" "placebo controlled" "prospective" studies are of higher quality than the "retrospective" reviews of previous treatments and results. I don't expect you to understand the ins and outs of research protocols; I just want you know that we "grade" the quality of the studies used to help *The G.A.I.N. Plan* evolve. Only the strongest evidence influences the suggestions made by *The G.A.I.N. Plan*. Since the science of health and longevity is in constant flux with new discoveries almost daily, The G.A.I.N. Plan is constantly evolving. This is why it is important to follow updates on our blogs and social media.

When it comes to your personal health, it is important to take the same approach that I take to my medical practice and the evolution of *G.A.I.N.* You need to take a step back periodically and objectively evaluate your progress. Although hard work is required for success, it is easy to "over-do it" or "under-do it" without objective evaluation.

When I was in my first year of bodybuilding competition, I thought I was training as hard as I could. To my surprise it wasn't until I hired a coach and had an objective opinion that I learned that I needed to train more focused on my weaknesses. I needed to increase the intensity of my cardiovascular exercise and eat more strictly. If you have a tendency to "under-do it" or lack the needed motivation to attain your goals, you will definitely find the tools of *The G.A.I.N. Plan* helpful. On the other hand, "over-doing it" can be to the detriment of the overzealous gym-goer leading to overtraining syndrome and/or chronic injury. Furthermore, there are clear signs proposed by *The G.A.I.N. Plan* to help you to avoid the overtraining syndrome.

Stress Your Health

Stress is a silent destroyer of all of your healthy intentions. Unlike the obvious problems of over indulgence, activity deficiency, and other bad habits, stress creeps up on you over time and sucks up your energy and well-being. You may not feel it while it's happening but once it reaches a certain threshold, the worst can happen.

Stress can be emotional, physical, mental, environmental, or any combination of these. Stress is a physical response to your environment and interpretation of your surroundings. Any circumstance in your life that invokes a need to respond with change, act unexpectedly, or regain balance can be considered stressful.

Stress can come in the form of negative or positive life events. For instance, a death in the family, trouble at work, natural disasters, being late for work and illness can all be considered negative life events. We won't perseverate on these because just thinking about them causes me stress. Positive life events that can invoke stress are moving to a new home, having a baby, starting a new job, entering into a new relationship. Even though these events seem like changes for the better, they are a change in your environment that requires readjustment of your way of life.

The Physiology of Stress

The G.A.I.N. Plan is all about building and maintaining muscle (anabolism) while limiting catabolism. Excessive stress is a destroyer of muscle; it is pure catabolism!

The "stress response" is an involuntary change in your body that comes with stressful life events. The response is related to the same "fight or flight" response that our ancient ancestors experienced to escape from their predators (i.e. the sabertooth tiger). In those days, the stress of the fight led to a need for bursts of energy to fight or run. This was a very physical response involving a series of physiological events in the body.

First, the perception of danger needs to occur. If you did not sense the danger of your attacker, there would be no need to jump into action.

This is a "decision" that you made via your cerebral cortex processing input from your senses. In some cases you may not be aware that you are making any decision, because the response is almost reflexive. This is especially true when the initial stimulus is pain. Second, your brain sends signals immediately to your body to do a number of things. Your muscles respond by putting you in motion. Your brain triggers the release of hormones from your hypothalamus to boost the stress hormones cortisol and epinephrine (adrenaline) from your adrenal glands. Cortisol has the ability to mobilize glucose into your blood in order to feed your brain and muscles during the fight or flight. Adrenalin and cortisol ramp up the whole system increasing heart rate, blood pressure, breathing, and concentration, resistance to pain, immunity, and strength. All of these responses were meant to occur for brief periods of time until you were able to escape danger. After the danger clears your body goes into a relaxation response where you recover from the stress with restoration of blood pressure and heart rate, normalization of digestive function, and calming of the mind for sleep.

Cortisol Effects:
- Controls blood glucose and insulin
- Regulates blood pressure
- Immune function
- Inflammatory response
- Shuts down non-essential functions like building bone, muscle, or skin

Although cortisol is essential for normal bodily functions, it is not meant to be elevated for long periods of time. Cortisol levels are highest in the morning after sleeping with an overnight fast. Cortisol helps to get you moving in the morning and maintains your blood glucose until you have breakfast. Its levels then follow a circadian pattern of slight elevations and depressions.

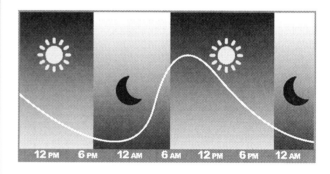

Fortunately, we do not frequently experience attacks by predators like our ancestors (unless you are defending our country, God Bless the Troops!). Unfortunately, we interpret many of our life situations much the same way as being attacked. We scream at other drivers on the road, we get frustrated with our bosses, we move non-stop from morning to night trying to cram 30 hours of work into a 24 hour day. With more of our stresses being psychological rather than physical, the physical responses to stress that still occur as they did in our ancestors' lead to problems in our bodies. We frequently delay the relaxation response for days, weeks, or even months. Those living in poverty may never have a relaxation response. This "chronic stress" causes chronic elevations in cortisol with significant consequences on our health.

Prolonged levels of cortisol result in system overload and exhaustion of many functions required for longevity and well-being. The overload results in:

1. Loss of muscle mass

2. Increase in body fat, especially in the midsection

3. Decreased immune function

4. Chronic inflammation damaging blood vessels and the brain

5. Impaired cognitive function: memory, concentration, and desire

6. Decreased bone density

7. High blood pressure, heart disease, and risk of stroke

8. Elevated blood glucose and potentially diabetes

9. Digestive and appetite dysfunction

10. Male and female hormonal imbalances

Chronic stress has been linked to many illnesses including early heart disease, dementia, and cancers. Some of this has to do with the effects of altered hormones like cortisol. Some stressors are related to the environment like "oxidative" stress from tissue damaging free radicals (*See Antioxidants). In animal studies stress results in cravings for unhealthy "comfort" foods that contribute to obesity, dyslipidemia, and diabetes.

Despite environmental stress, the majority of the physical effects of stress come from the perception of our environment. Your boss walking into your office can be a stressful event if you have the misconception that he is out to fire you. If your attitude is predominantly negative, you are likely to think this way. Otherwise, he might just be checking in to say hi. Although the major emotional stressors in life, like a divorce or a death, cause noticeable physical distress in the form of depression, fatigue, tearfulness, etc most of the stressors we experience are not as obvious. It is often difficult to realize just how much stress you are under until you take a step back and analyze your situation. What you will likely find is that most of your stressors are self-induced.

Your Own Signs of Stress

People react to stress in very different ways. The first thing you need to do is identify your own signs of stress. This will allow you to recognize the early warning signs that you are getting stressed out. This is like that dummy light in your car. When the dummy oil light goes on and you ignore it, instead of paying for a few quarts of oil, you'll will shortly end up needing a new car.

You should look for 4 kinds of stress signs:

- Those affecting physical health or bodily functions:
  - Back/Neck Pain or muscle tension, Upset stomach, sweaty, chest tight/changes in breathing, fatigue, frequent urination, palpitations, sweaty palms

- Those affecting your feelings:
  - Sad, mad, irritable, worried, anxious, or tense

- Those affecting your behavior:
  - Sleep more or less, eat more or less, fidgety, restless legs, use drugs/tobacco, less libido, impulsive

- Those affecting your thoughts:
  - Lack of concentration, memory deficits, loss of optimism, helpless/hopeless thoughts

Go through each one of these kinds of stress and pick a symptom that fits how you become under stress. Learning to recognize when you are experiencing these will act as your "dummy light" for the times to get some stress management. Remember to employ healthy relaxation and recovery techniques to avoid falling into the spiral of frustration and despair. We will go over a few of these in the section Address Your Stress.

Ideally, we should just get away from stressful situations.Unfortunately, too often we just can't do that. However we can learn to control our response to stressful situations. Once you figure out what your stressors are you can decide if your responses to those stressors are appropriate. This will reduce the effects of stress on your mental and physical health.

Try writing down the major stressors in your life:

1. Physical (i.e. smoking, lack of sleep, pain, overeating, lack of veggies, etc):

   _____

   _____

2. Mental (i.e. exams, deadlines, projects, money, work):

_____

_____

3. Emotional (i.e. relationships, social situations):

_____

_____

Take a look at these stressors closely and see if any of these are only stressors because of "thought distortions" (see list in "ATTITUDE"). For those that don't seem to be thought distortions, write out ways to *address the stress*. Just the act of writing these down may invoke physical feelings of stress related to these issues. Listen to your breathing, heart rate, and stomach. Are you getting a tight feeling in your stomach or chest? Are you holding your breath more? Are you having trouble concentrating after thinking of one of these issues?

Some people are at higher risk for the negative physical effects of stress than others. Your occupation may be more stressful than others. For instance, being a firefighter is a very stressful job. However, you may be a "type A" personality that demands perfection and attention to detail in an otherwise less stressful job. This is not necessarily a bad thing. What you need to realize is that if you have a more stressful job than others or if you are an anxious "type A" you need to spend more time working on the recovery response to stress.

As I write this section, I am conjuring up stressful issues in my own life. As I do this I am stopping to write them down. It is very cathartic. If I don't write them down they are just ethereal and can continue to disrupt more productive thinking. Writing down your stressors makes them concrete and addressable.

Address Your Stress

Stress Relaxation Techniques

Some forms of stress in everyday life are going to be there no matter what we do. The best way to deal with this type of stress is to recognize it and change your perspective on the event. For instance, if you are constantly held up in traffic try listening to an audio book or start authoring your own book on a Dictaphone. Turn a bad situation into a productive one.

Once you have recognized how your mind and body respond to stress spend some time writing a stress log. Each day for a week, write down time and date whenever your stress dummy light goes off. After a week review the list. The act of doing this may help you realize that there are proactive ways to avoid the stress. For instance, you may realize that all you need to do is arrive and leave work 15 minutes earlier and you'll cut your commute in half. It may also impress your boss that you are the first one in each day.

When your dummy light goes on, your body is already responding with the "fight or flight" response. To nip it in the bud, you can try a few techniques on the next pages.

1. PAY ATTENTION TO YOUR BREATHING.

When we are under stress we have a tendency to hold our breath, chest breath, and take shorter breaths. Stop and take some deep breaths counting 5 seconds in and 5 seconds out. Also, do this through your belly by expanding it on the way in and squeezing on the way out. Try this for 10 breaths.

2. SMILE.

Take a step back and think of whether your face is tense. Do you have a frown? Is your brow scrunched up? Try to relax the muscles of your face and then try to generate a genuine smile. Think of something funny. Make a concerted effort to tell someone a joke. Keep a funny picture of your kids or pets in your wallet. If you aren't able to step out of a stressful situation, put on a smile anyway. It will make you appear less confrontational with whomever you encounter.

3. TIME OUT.

If it is possible to take some time for you just do it! It could be just as simple as closing your eyes and counting to 10.

4. THOUGHT CONTROL.

Recognize your stressful feelings and thoughts and just hit the pause button. Stop your stressful thoughts before you begin perseverating on them. Think of positives in your life or situation. Practice mindfulness and look for the empty space between thoughts that free you from judgment.

These techniques will help you for when you
recognize that you are under stress. But, just as
in medicine an ounce of prevention is worth a
pound of cure. Through proper exercise, sleep,
nutrition, and active rest you will manage your
physical and mental stress before it gets out
of control.

Overtraining and The Athlete Triad

For some the thought of overtraining might
seem like a joke, as so many of us are relatively
sedentary already. This is not something that
you should skip over though. Any time you move
from one level of activity to another of greater
activity, you have the risk of adding too much
stress too soon or too often (The Terrible Too's).
In fact, simply trying a new exercise can lead
to excess stress on an unaccustomed. Thus, it
is important for you to recognize the signs and
symptoms of overtraining.

Training is a process of overload that is meant
to disturb balance in the body (homeostasis).
It results in acute fatigue and muscle soreness,
but leads to improvements in performance.
Sometimes you might throw in a couple weeks
of high intensity training, like a training camp.
Because of the prolonged high intensity nature
of this type of training there is almost always
a short-term performance decrement. With
some active rest after such intense training, you
can reap improvements in performance. This
short burst of intense training is referred to as
"functional overreaching".

Functional overreaching is a short-term
period of high intensity training that leads to a

brief drop in performance anticipating a greater return with planned recovery afterward.

If you do not respect the stressful effects of the intense training on your body's physiology and skip the recovery period, you do more harm than good. This is called *"nonfunctional" overreaching* and is very similar to ignoring other forms of stress in how it affects your body. Not only do you begin to experience muscular fatigue and weakness, but psychological distress and hormonal imbalances occur. When your training reaches this exhaustive stage, if you persist and fail to *"address your stress"*, *overtraining syndrome* occurs. Overtraining syndrome can lead to career ending injuries, desire to quit your sport or activity, and can take months to recover from once finally recognized.

To keep things simple, think of overreaching this way. Earlier we discussed training to be done with 2 steps forward with an expected 1 step back. This is "training" with steady progress. Sometimes the system needs a little shock to break through barriers and overcome plateaus. Functional overreaching is 4 steps forward and 2 to 3 steps back utilized when trying to break through a plateau. If you don't allow for recovery and continue with 5, 6, or 7 steps forward you may get to the dreaded overtraining syndrome.

Recognizing Overtraining Syndrome

Overtraining Syndrome (OTS) is a condition affecting your mind and body that occurs when your exercise volume and intensity exceed your recuperative capacity. It is one of exceedingly diminishing returns. The physical aspects are related to over-expenditure of energy, a lack of available nutrients, and insufficient rest. Chronic stressors in the form of emotions, learned behaviors, social stress, and even addiction can perpetuate the recovery debt that leads to OTS.

OTS RESULTS IN SYMPTOMS OF:

- persistent muscle soreness
- weakness
- lack of endurance
- fatigue
- decreased immune function with respiratory illness
- irritability and depression
- loss of appetite
- loss of motivation
- sleep disturbances

MEASURABLE SIGNS OF OVERTRAINING SYNDROME INCLUDE:

- lower white blood cell count
- weight loss
- increased resting heart rate (heart rate when sleeping)
- decreased strength
- increased submaximal heart rate (goes higher while doing less)
- lower anabolic hormone levels (testosterone, GH) and higher cortisol levels
- changes in menstrual cycle (women)
- erectile dysfunction (men)

ASK YOURSELF:

- Does exercise exhaust you instead of invigorate you?
- Do you feel blue or down in the dumps?
- Are you unable to sleep or have un-restful sleep?
- Do you get sick easily or have trouble getting over colds?
- Do your legs just feel "heavy"?
- Do you have a short fuse?
- Is your muscle soreness taking longer to go away than before?

Overtraining may occur because of a poorly planned workout routine or a schedule that doesn't allow for adequate recovery. This could mean that an exercise is repeated too often or the intensity on repeated bouts is too high. It may occur during periods of increasing training volume or intensity compounded by social or environmental stress. Overtraining is more likely to occur when an athlete is exposed to other psychological and physical stressors like travel, relationship problems, school work, employment, or family problems. *As we discussed earlier in Attitude, traumatic experiences only improve resiliency and performance when adequate time is given to recover from the added stress. Otherwise, stress accumulates and a break down in the system occurs whereas the athlete loses the ability to perform.

The physiological explanations for overtraining syndrome include many overlapping theories. First, micro-trauma to muscles occurs during training. When micro-trauma is created faster than the body can heal it, they become cumulative in the form of an injury. Second, relative caloric or protein deficiency occurs. When the body is trying to recover from exercise it needs consistent supplies of protein. The American College of Sports Medicine suggests that athletes need to consume more protein than the average population to recover and grow after exercise. If energy supplies are deficient the body will break down muscle as an energy source. This is completely counterproductive to your performance goals. Third, the body ends up in a catabolic state with elevated stress hormones like cortisol and lower anabolic hormones like testosterone or growth hormone. Fourth, excessive psychological and physical strain results in fatigue of the central nervous system. Fatigue of the central nervous system is closely tied to muscle weakness, immune dysfunction, disordered thinking (depression and lack of concentration), decreased tolerance of exertion, and impaired sleep.

If overtraining is not recognized and addressed early in the plateau of performance, you will suffer a decline in performance that can be goal threatening. Muscular and mental fatigue results in poor decision making in training and loss of technique in performance of your discipline. In technique intensive activities like gymnastics, dance, or ski jumping, failure of technique can have catastrophic consequences. As I described in the beginning of the book, recovery debt, a stressful job, and lack of sleep led to my catastrophic bicep tendon tear. Further, loss of core strength can cause back injuries. Loss of agility can cause non-contact knee injuries. Loss of balance control can cause falls. Successful athletes spend much of their off season on improving core strength, agility, and balance to reduce the risk of injury. Studies support their efforts.

The Overtraining Triad

One form of overtraining that is of great interest to clinicians and researchers is the "female athlete triad". This is a phenomenon that is characterized by:

1.   Disordered eating

2.   Amenorrhea

3.   Lower bone density

This is a problem that was initially described in women who overtrained and had energy deficits from eating too little. As a result their performance declined along with their bone density. When bone density declines these athletes become at risk for debilitating stress fractures. I would like to suggest here that this is not a triad unique only to females. Males can suffer from the same problem. The bone density problem may not be the biggest issue, but a loss of lean body mass (muscle) correlates well with loss of bone mineral density in many studies. So to re-define the "Over-training Triad" for men and women:

1.   Low nutrient availability

2.   Hormonal imbalance

3.   Diminished lean body mass

It is important to note that once the hormonal imbalance and loss of lean mass occurs, the horse is already out of the barn. Now it's time to play catch up, while losing precious training

time. Hopefully, you have recognized your overtraining and lack of recovery before this occurs.
Because of the label "female" athlete triad, the
problems that occur in the overtrained male
have been relatively overlooked. However, data
on females shows that effective nutritional
interventions are needed to improve dietary
intakes and eating behaviors of college athletes.
For example one study found that 91% of
collegiate female athletes failed to eat enough
calories to support their training, 36% consumed
less than 5 meals per day, and the majority of
participants failed to eat a regular breakfast
or monitor their hydration status. *These are
statistics that make it imperative that we spread
the word of G.A.I.N. to college coaches.

Men and women have statistically different
issues with food. Studies support that female
athletes are more likely to restrict calories and
use diet supplements than male athletes out of
concerns about body fat. Men tend to be more
interested in muscle size, strength, and speed
than body fat. The deficiency that occurs in men
is more likely to be related to a lack of nutrient
availability for their goals. For instance, if the
male athlete partakes in high volume endurance
training with two-a-day workouts and a rigorous
course load at school, they may not have time
to consume enough carbohydrate or protein to
maintain their muscle recovery. They may also
lack supportive nutrients like a multivitamin and
become relatively micronutrient deficient. The
result in both males and females is that the lack
of nutrients causes incomplete recovery from
training. In the worst case scenario, both men
and women can suffer from clinical problems

such as anorexia nervosa (lack of eating/over exercising) or bulimia (binge and purge) leading to the overtraining triad.

Fortunately, even in the worst case scenarios of severe anorexia where the body goes into survival mode with kidney problems, bone marrow dysfunction, irregular heartbeat, and cognitive impairment, the body has an incredible ability to regenerate. In order to recover, nutrient intake must exceed the nutrient minimum for balancing energy output and input. No matter the level of activity, if energy output exceeds energy input the body goes into starvation survival mode. Switching on "survival mode" causes slowing of metabolism, decreases in anabolic hormones, an increase in catabolic hormones, and increased use of stored fats and muscle for energy. Human physiology exists such that the brain must always have fuel. The brain dictates the breakdown of vital parts of the body to maintain a constant supply of energy.

Unfortunately, the line between overreaching and overtraining syndrome is quite vague. In essence, when your training causes not only persistent decrease in your performance, but you experience significant mental duress (depression, fatigue, frustration), then you are likely in nonfunctional overreaching or overtraining syndrome.

In order to understand the evolution of the overtraining syndrome it is important to rule out concomitant medical and environmental stressors that when left unaddressed leave you at risk for persistent loss of performance.

1. Negative energy balance
2. Lack of essential amino acid or fats
3. Magnesium, iron, vitamin D, potassium deficiency
4. Food and environmental allergies
5. Hypothyroidism, Insulin resistance, Hypogonadism
6. Infections
7. Toxic exposures including smoking, alcohol, and drugs
8. Dehydration and cold/heat stress
9. Sleep disorders
10. Unrecognized psychiatric illness or chemical imbalances

The biggest challenge presented to *The G.A.I.N. Plan* is development of methods to assess training progress while detecting the start overtraining syndrome before it becomes disabling. Blood work has been suggested to look for markers of overtraining syndrome. Some have suggested that lactic acid elevations, falls in glutamine levels, and decreased heart rate variability correlate with the onset of overtraining. However, these tests are very inconsistent across studies and have little value to the athlete in day to day training. So the athlete and *G.A.I.N. Planner* need to recognize the effects of OTS on performance and attitude.

1. PERFORMANCE LEVELS

Decreases in performance can be detected by performing the "standardized exercise test" (see Fatigue in ATTITUDE). Having a baseline test is critical to further evaluation. Decreases in performance can often be more closely detected by having a sport specific measure of performance that you perform on a periodic basis. Pick an activity like the bench press. Pick a weight that you can perform 10 reps to failure. Use this weight as a baseline. If you find it harder to do than your previous workout, you probably haven't recovered enough or you took too much time off. You can do this with a mile run, the rowing machine, or any other consistent activity. *Use the ratings of perceived exertion and heart rate with these tests as your perceived exertion may be affected by attitude changes.

2.   ATTITUDE CHANGES

The presence of psychological symptoms in overtraining is clearly a defining factor of the syndrome, but often difficult to detect. The psychological effects of intense training can present themselves prior to the physiological effects and thus present a unique monitoring opportunity to avoid overtraining. Measures of fatigue and vigor are even more sensitive than that of depression until overtraining is reached. In a state of overtraining depressive symptoms of lack of concentration, hopelessness, appetite changes and sleep disturbances prevail. *In the implementation section of this book there is a simple quiz to assess your physical and mental readiness to train hard. Also, there are more in-depth POMS (perception of moods states) questionnaires at www.yourgainplan.com.

The key to these psychological tests is honesty. Sometimes the mood disturbance itself changes your attitude toward the testing. Sometimes you may be tempted to "fake" good or bad to manipulate your own program. Honesty and integrity are virtues that will help you in life at all levels and lead to longevity. You must start with being honest with yourself. *The G.A.I.N. Plan* will only be of value to you in improving your performance if you are honest in your input data.

3. BIOMETRIC MEASUREMENTS

Your resting heart rate, heart rate recovery, and heart rate response to exercise can give you some objective measures of your training progress. As you become more cardiovascularly fit your resting heart rate declines. Professional endurance athletes can have remarkably low resting heart rates. If you are overtraining, you may notice a persistent rise in your resting heart rate. Also, when you are overtrained, your heart rate recovers more slowly after exercise as it must work harder under the added stress. Further, your heart rate may rise faster and stay more elevated at the start of exercise causing a feeling of increased exertion.   This is where your perceived exertion tests are also elevated.

Measuring your activity level throughout the day with an actigraph (accelerometer) can give you an accurate assessment of your caloric expenditure. ombining this with measures of heart rate can improve the accuracy of the measurement. By recording your caloric intake through recall or a scheduled diet you can compare your intake vs expenditure. If you notice persistent excessive expenditure beyond a 500 calorie deficit per day (maximum allowed by G.A.I.N. for 1 lb per week weight loss) take heed that you may be treading the path to overtraining.

Overcoming Overtraining

For those that have difficulty with getting motivated and just getting to the gym, you may not think that "over-training" could ever pertain to you. This would be misguided thinking. The novice athlete or gym-goer is probably at the highest risk for Over-Training syndrome. Once you acquire the desire to be in the gym, the tendency is for the "more is better" mentality to take over. More weight, more reps, more days in the gym does not always equate to more progress. I learned this the hard way, so you don't have to. However, the desire to complete the CCC and "join the club" may push you to new levels.

Before you become accustomed to how a particular training regimen will affect your body over the next couple days, it is important to take your time with your exercise progression. Graded exercise applies to not only the gradual "grade" to your increased intensity and "grading" of your progress, but also "grading" your physiologic and mental state between and before workouts. If you are remarkably sore the day after a workout it doesn't make sense that you train the same way again the next day or even at the next session of the same body part. Persistent stress on your body and the pain it produces will lead to detriments in muscle recovery and attitudes toward future workouts (fear, skepticism, lack of interest).

For competitive athletes, many begin to approach overtraining just a few weeks before major competitions as training is ramped up. However, an experienced athlete or coach will realize that the important work is done in the month before the competition and not the couple weeks before. Thus, the density (reps, sets, and rest periods) and intensity of workouts goes through a taper in the last couple weeks before a competition. This taper allows for physiologic recovery at the muscle, cardiac, endocrine, and nervous system levels. The body is allowed to adapt and recover from the intense training and the athlete will be able to functionally "over-reach" at the competition.

Training density: The time lag between training stimuli during and between workouts. This includes the number of workout days per week (and thus rest days also), the number of exercises, sets (intervals in HIIT), reps or per workout and the rest you take between sets.

For some, being in the gym every day of the week is a necessary stress reliever and is just ingrained in their routine. This is certainly the case for me. However, if I train at 110% intensity every day I know that I will do more harm than good. To do this safely you must vary between low, moderate, and high intensity workouts or split up body parts by training a well-rested body part from day to day. You should not be doing full body workouts each day or HIIT every day. With insufficient rest (including sleep and nutrition) cortisol levels will rise and anabolic hormones will cease production. Reductions in anabolic hormones like testosterone result in further fatigue, muscle weakness, muscle atrophy, depressive symptoms, and lack of libido.

If you find that you are knee deep in overtraining syndrome try some of the principles on the next pages.

Principles for Overcoming Overtraining:

1. CUT YOUR WORKOUTS DOWN TO 3 DAYS PER WEEK AT MOST.

    You may need to do this for a couple weeks to a month depending on how deep of a recovery deficit you have accumulated Again, this really is relative rest. Activities like LISS cardio or stretching can still be performed in most situations up to 5 days per week. However, if all you were doing is LISS cardio when you discovered the over-training, you may need to scale it back further to just stretching or physical therapy type exercises.

2. DECREASE YOUR INTENSITY AND DENSITY IN THE GYM.

    You can increase rest periods between sets, lift lighter, or go back to basic exercises that your muscle is very familiar with. By avoiding new or complex exercises, you can give your muscle a chance to recover and avoid worsening of delayed onset muscle soreness (which occurs commonly after introducing new exercises). You can watch your heart rate to avoid significant elevations (i.e. >65% HR_{max} during recovery workouts. Avoid super sets and circuits to allow for more recovery time. Also avoid taking your sets to failure. You should feel as though you can comfortably complete 2-3 more repetitions without breaking form.

    Avoid the intensity increasing techniques we discussed earlier, like assisted reps, drop sets, and cheat reps. Besides using your heart rate you can use a stopwatch to time a

90-120 second rest between sets to avoid the tendency to inadvertently increase intensity.

3. MAKE SURE THAT CALORIES CONSUMED ARE MORE THAN CALORIES BURNED.

It is very important that when you are in a potentially over-trained state that you are fueling the body for recovery. Added protein and carbohydrate may be necessary to overcome nutritional deficiencies. It is important to adjust your training volume, intensity, and density to avoid exceeding your caloric intake in energy expenditure. It is this energy deficit that drives the metabolic and hormonal dysfunction in overtraining syndrome. If your goal has been to lose weight, you may have to go back to eating neutral or positive calories for a week or two to restore homeostasis.

4. PERFORM SOME RECREATIONAL RECOVERY.

By participating in some recreational low intensity sports like golfing, bowling, or doubles tennis you can break from the regular training routine and rejuvenate the soul at the same time with a little fun. You will rest your brain from any repetition that you had fallen into with your regular exercise routine.

5. REDUCE IMPACT

Neuromuscular fatigue is a serious over-training issue. Your joints and muscles provide constant feed back to the motor centers of your brain in order to produce reflexive responses to agility challenges.

If this system is fatigued, the reflexes may be slowed or disordered resulting in joint instability and higher risk for injury. Go back to basics during your recovery time and work on re-training these reflexes in a controlled fashion (i.e. ACL prevention drills, balance, and proprioceptive exercises).

6.   RE-ASSESS YOUR GOALS AND PREPARE FOR FUTURE INCREASES IN TRAINING INTENSITY.

Visualize where you want to be in a month, a year, or 10 years from now. Realization that everything doesn't have to be done right now is critical to long-term longevity and success in life and sport. Remember how to eat an elephant? Decide what is important to you. Write a plan down.Grade yourself and keep track of progress. Tell others and make some accountability in your social network.

7.   MONITOR HR (*SEE GRADED EXCERCISE)

Look for restoration or improvement in your baseline resting heart rate. Test yourself with the Standardized exercise test that you created at the start of your plan. Through graded techniques you will always have a baseline of yesterday's self.

The Importance of Sleep

Sleep is the time when both your body and mind get to recuperate. Disordered sleep with difficulty falling to sleep, frequent awakenings, restless sleep activity, and low quantity are all signs of stressors and actually add more stress to the situation. Sometimes sleep can be the cause of over-training syndrome and lack of recovery such as when you are under a great deal of emotional or work related stress. Disordered sleep itself can be a sign of overtraining manifesting from endocrine and nervous system dysfunction.

From a medical perspective, if you notice that you are having excessive day time sleepiness, wake often during the night, have snoring issues, or you are having upper respiratory issues it is possible that you may be dealing with obstructive sleep apnea (OSA). OSA is characterized by repetitive pauses in breathing during sleep, despite the effort to breathe.In OSA, the pauses in breathing, which are called "apneas" typically last 20 to 40 seconds. During the apneas the oxygen in your blood drops and can cause further issues due to lack of oxygen. Often, your significant other or family members will notice these episodes before you ever do. If you are having problems of this sort and especially excessive daytime sleepiness, it is very important to bring this up with your primary care physician. OSA can lead to significant systemic illness, higher risk for early death from other illness, and even sleep episodes during driving or operating machinery which can be damaging to you, your property, and others.

To understand how the quality of sleep affects your body's recovery and metabolism it is important to explain the "architecture" of healthy sleep. Sleep occurs in a series of stages and goes through a number of cycles of those stages throughout a night of sleep.

Much like a workout with weights, sleep involves multiple sets with varying intensities. Consider sleep to be an "active" recuperation process.

Sleep follows a pattern that alternates between two types of sleep: REM (rapid eye movement) and Non-REM sleep (NREM). NREM makes up approximately 75% of sleep and consists of 3 stages (the classic 3rd and 4th can be considered as one stage).

Stage 1 (N1): Light sleep, the border between being awake and falling asleep; drowsy, muscle jerks, and hallucination like occurrences

Stage 2 (N2): Onset of sleep, conscious awareness of the external environment ceases; muscles relax and body temperature drops.

Stage 3 (N3): This is considered deep or "slow wave sleep"; this is when most of the restorative effects of sleep occur; growth hormone is released.

REM Sleep: "rapid eye movement"; 25% of the sleep cycle; REM occur after the first 90 minutes of sleep and then again every 90 minutes, as the night goes on the REM stage gets longer; this is a state very close to wakening but muscles are completely relaxed (somewhat paralyzed); dreams occur during REM; it is thought that memories are consolidated during this stage.

Sleep progresses in cycles of REM and NREM, with up to four or five of them per night. The order of sleep stages is normally N1 → N2 → N3 → N2 →REM. More of deep sleep (N3) occurs earlier in the night, while the proportion of REM sleep increases in the cycles just before natural awakening.

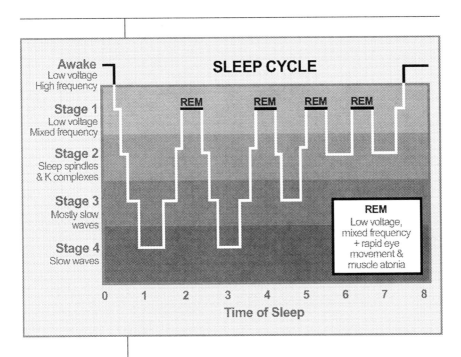

If this pattern is disrupted you can imagine that you might spend less time in the restorative N3 sleep. Monitoring your sleep can be performed via electroencephalograms (which are costly) or via monitoring of body motion. N3 and REM sleep are thought to be the most important stages for recuperative effects of sleep and are the stages where you are most immobile. The more active you are during sleep, the potentially less restorative your sleep is for your body and mind.

Of course, in our busy lives we must make a conscious effort to get on a regular sleep schedule. Even the best intentioned sleeper will have a night where they lose a little sleep; studying or working on a project. As long as you do not make a habit of limiting your sleep and accumulating sleep debt you can have a night like this now and then. Try to avoid more than 2

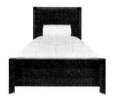

days of limited sleep. Accumulation of sleep debt over 4 to 5 days has proven detrimental effects on hormones and metabolism. Getting some extra sleep after a few days of deprivation is ok, but returning to a routine of 7 to 9 hours of sleep is critical to staying anabolic. Remember, sleep is not being lazy and unproductive; it is actively recovering and rejuvenating your body and mind.

Some Tips for a Good Night Sleep:

1. GET IN A ROUTINE:

    Establish a regular bed time and wake time and stick to it as close as possible. Keep a regular waking time. Even if you go to bed late, get up at the same time every day. Your body runs on a biological clock that starts each morning when you open your eyes. If you sleep longer the clock starts later and you may have trouble going to sleep the following night.

2. AVOID STIMULANTS:

    Avoid taking any stimulants within 4 to 5 hours of bed time. If you are having insomnia issues, avoid stimulants all together.

3. AVOID ALCOHOL AND OTC SLEEP AIDS:

    Alcohol can disrupt your sleep architecture and result in less restorative sleep; other sleep aids can be addicting and lead to bad habits and residual sleepiness upon waking.

4. AVOID EXERCISING TOO CLOSE TO BED TIME:

    Getting your heart rate and body temperature up before bed time can be disruptive to healthy sleep.

5. "WIND-DOWN":

   Get into the habit of dropping projects or studying with a period of relaxation (i.e. a recreational book, meditation, or visualization) prior to bed time.

6. BUILD YOUR CAVE:

   Some effort needs to be put into where you hibernate. You need a comfortable bed, pillow, and sheets. Make the room as dark and quiet as possible with curtains and ear plugs if necessary.

7. THE BED IS FOR SLEEP AND SEX:

   Remove distractions like a TV, computers, cell phones. The bedroom is for sleeping not working and socializing with Facebook friends. The light from phones and computers can affect your brain's response to night time. Stop using these devices at least an hour before bed.

8. SET THE THERMOSTAT:

   Most people find it difficult to sleep in a hot room, but just be sure that the temperature suits your own level of comfort.

9. IF YOU WAKE UP IN THE NIGHT:

   Get out of bed, go to a chair, have a glass of milk and read a little; don't lay in bed staring at the ceiling.

10. NEVER GO TO BED ANGRY:

    Whether you are married or not this is good advice; if you fought with someone in the home, swallow your pride and apologize. If you are angry at others, try to forgive and forget. See the positives of any interaction in life.

Supplements for Sleep

1. L-TRYPTOPHAN:

    This is a sedating amino acid found in the diet that has some controversy behind it. Supplemented L-tryptophan (4-5g/day) increases brain levels of the amino acid and where it acts as a precursor for the neurotransmitter serotonin. In doing so, it causes drowsiness that is useful for initiating sleep. In 1989, the use of L-tryptophan supplements was linked to a syndrome with severe muscle pain and elevated eosinophil counts in the blood dubbed "eosinophilia myalgia syndrome". As it turned out, the syndrome appeared to be caused by a contaminant from production and not from the L-tryptophan itself.

2. KAVA KAVA:

    This is a preparation from the plant Piper methysticum which contains six psychoactive "kavalactones". These compounds bind to GABA receptors (like benzodiazepines), dopamine receptors, and opiod receptors leading to reductions in anxiety symptoms. Numerous studies support that Kava has the ability to improve anxiety related insomnia. The Kava Anxiety Depression Spectrum Study was a 3-week placebo-controlled, double-blind study supplementing with 250 mg of kavalactones per day. The study showed significant improvement in anxiety symptoms and appeared safe. However, the FDA has previously issued a warning that Kava supplements may disrupt liver metabolism of medications and potentially cause liver toxicity. You may want to think twice about this supplement if you are using liver toxic drugs.

3. VALERIAN ROOT

This is a temperate root and has been in use since the time of Hippocrates. Valerian root appears to increase synthesis of GABA and thus has sedative and anti-anxiety effects, When taken at doses of 400–900 mg daily valerian root is as effective as diazepam (Valium) in reducing psychiatric rating scales of anxiety. A randomized triple blinded placebo controlled study in 2011 demonstrated that 530mg of concentrated valerian extract significantly improved quality of sleep in women with insomnia.

4. L-THEANINE

This is an amino acid found in green tea with anti-anxiety effects that can help with going to sleep. L-theanine produces a calming effect on the brain by crossing the blood-brain barrier and increasing the production of both GABA and dopamine. In a clinical study, subjects were given 200mg of L-theanine or a benzodiazepine and subjected to experimentally induced anxiety. The people who received L-theanine had significantly lower baseline anxiety.

5.   MELATONIN

This is a natural hormone released by the pineal gland in the brain that helps regulate the sleep-wake cycle (circadian rhythms) by transmitting information about light and dark to the body. I have written extensively on melatonin as as its effects are numerous and span the spectrum of anti-oxidant, anti-cancer, anabolic, and immune effects. Melatonin can help you fall asleep through its sedating effects and improve the restorative effects of sleep. Prolonged-Release formulations of melatonin may even help in cases where you tend to wake up in the middle of the night. Melatonin is usually taken at doses of 3 to 5mg. Melatonin can even be effective for jet lag if taken on the day of departure at the bed time of your destination and a few days thereafter before bed.

Massage and Recovery

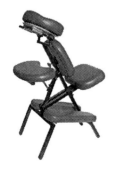

Who doesn't like a good massage? If you have ever had a therapeutic massage you know it can have powerful effects. When you walk into the clinic and lay on the table you can just feel the weight of the world being pulled, kneaded, and rubbed right off your body. When you walk out your legs feel like Gumby and your head feels lighter with your neck sporting appreciable suppleness. It's a fantastic feeling, similar to the satisfaction one gets after a hard workout in the gym.

Despite the fact that massage therapy is a 10 to 11 billion dollar industry with up to 10% of the American population partaking in treatments every year, there are skeptics to its validity and usefulness in healthcare. The reason for this may be that the evidence to support the beneficial effects of massage therapy had been very unreliable and lacked scientific scrutiny until recent years. Massage therapy has always been labeled an "alternative" treatment along with acupuncture, chiropractic care, and mindfulness techniques. This goes along with the fact that the science to support the clinical and cost effectiveness of these disciplines is not typically as robust as current evidenced-based medical practice. Many of these disciplines have been around for centuries and are just accepted as useful based on the fact that they have withstood the test of time.

With regards to massage therapy and studying its physiological effects and clinical effectiveness, there are many techniques and variables that make standardization difficult. Massage may be the oldest existing medical treatment dating back to >2000 years BC. Ancient Greek and Indian texts describe massage as a therapy for treating sports and war injuries. It was used widely by Hippocrates and the Roman Empire. The social decadence of massage and the "happy ending" tarnished the reputation of massage until the late 1800s, when new techniques sprouted and scientific research began to explore its effectiveness. Many different techniques varying in pressure applied, use of tools, patterns of application, and frequency of use have evolved over the centuries.

Scientific evidence supports how various techniques improve muscle and blood vessel physiology and some are better than others at affecting different aspects of tissue biology.

Massage dilates superficial blood vessels and increases the rate of blood flow via local nerve mediated reflexes. Forceful massage even increases the amount of blood volume pumped out of the heart by improving venous return. Flow rates may take up to 1 hour to return to normal after a deep tissue massage. With these effects on blood flow this data suggests that massage may be able to improve muscle performance and recovery.

Recent data supports that massage therapy can possibly enhance recovery from exercise. In the well-respected journal, *Science Translational Medicine*, researchers demonstrated that massage therapy to the quadriceps after exercise-induced muscle damage resulted in reductions of inflammation and improved energy efficiency. The researchers noted that despite having no effect on muscle lactate or glycogen, massage decreased inflammatory markers thus countering the cellular stress produced with muscle injury. Interestingly, they also found a rise in "mitochondrial biogenesis" which may have the benefit of improving energy production in subsequent bouts of exercise. Unfortunately for us, this research did not include follow up on strength, muscle growth, endurance, or performance.

Of particular note, the fable that "lactic acid is massaged out of the muscle" has been disproven in multiple studies including the above study.

Although massage after painful exercise makes sense for improving pain and recovery, what about its use before exercise? The use of massage before, during, and after sporting events has become quite popular. If you watched the London Olympics you saw a number of scenes where athletes were being probed and kneaded while lying on rows of tables. But is this really helpful?

Psychologically, there is good evidence that massage has a calming effect and may help athletes who require steady nerves and intense concentration or fine motor control. However, research published in 2011 in the *Journal of Strength and Conditioning Research* showed that pre-event massage resulted in a calming response that correlated with a decrease in muscle performance. Thus I would suggest that pre-event massage be limited to sports that require fine motor skill and those events which benefit from a reduction in nervous tension.

Studies of the effects of massage on your general health have shown real potential for medical efficacy. The systemic effects of massage include a dose dependent response with twice weekly Swedish massage raising oxytocin (a pleasure hormone) levels and decreasing cortisol levels. The acute effects of massage in healthy individuals include a rise in white cell immune response. This implies a possible increase in resistance to illness like colds and flu.

Swedish massage may have a more beneficial effect on lowering blood pressure than more vigorous techniques like sports massage and trigger point therapy which may actually increase blood pressure. There is support that massage can improve mood and anxiety while decreasing cortisol levels that are elevated by stress. Swedish massage also works well in the treatment of osteoarthritis of the knee resulting in improvements in pain scores and walking distance. Many other studies support the use of massage therapy in the treatment of low back pain, cancer pain, Parkinson's disease, fibromyalgia, and Morton's neuroma. Although the quality of the research is quite variable, the lack of downsides of massage other than the cost suggests it could be used in these otherwise difficult to treat conditions.

The nice thing about massage is that is can be done just about anywhere. If you don't have a therapist or a partner that can help you, there are many devices that are available on the market. One of the simplest tools for self-massage is the foam roller. Foam rollers have become very popular in recent years and can be used to perform self-myofascial release. Rollers that are more firm or have multilevel rigidity can apply more consistent pressure and may be more effective. A study at the Memorial University of New Foundland published in the *Journal of Strength and Conditioning Research* in May of 2012 demonstrated that foam roller self-myofascial release applied to the quadriceps improved range of motion without any concomitant deficit in muscle performance. Myofascial release techniques can improve parasympathetic outflow after exercise and thus help heart rate recovery and return to normal blood pressure.

Massage therapy is quite popular and has been around for centuries. It has probably persisted in our culture because it has real effects on our psychology and physiology. The euphoric feelings that it can produce when done well by a therapist can be addicting.With its immune-modulatory effects and reduction in stress hormone levels massage has clear benefits to your longevity. Look for a certified massage therapist who is respected in your community, and avoid those places with $5 "happy endings".

No Pain, No G.A.I.N.?

I hope you have already appreciated the importance of recovery and injury prevention in pursuit of your G.A.I.N. Plan. Pain is a normal response to physical stress. However, all pains are not created equal. Notably, especially for the novice athlete it may not be as clear as to when pain is due to muscle soreness versus injury. In this section we will give you some tips on recognizing the difference.

Delayed Onset Muscle Soreness (DOMS) and The "Burn"

Otherwise known as *"DOMS"*, delayed onset muscle soreness is pain and stiffness in muscle groups that have been exposed to strenuous exercise, especially exercise to which the muscle is unaccustomed. The soreness which usually evolves within 24 to 72 hours after the exercise involves a healing process that leads to muscle adaptations to exercise including getting bigger and stronger. The pain is often a dull aching that occurs with touching the muscle or with movement.

Eccentric exercise (the negative) where the muscle is lengthening while contracting, such as lowering a weight down slowly, will more likely result in DOMS. Muscles adapt quickly to this type of exercise making repeated bouts less likely to result in DOMS. Training "the negative" can be a very effective, but painful way to build muscle. Stretching, massage, and lighter activity are recommended to relieve the discomfort.

DOMS is not the same as "*the burn*" that occurs during exercise. The burn, often thought to be from a buildup of lactic acid in the muscle, is where the concept "No pain, no gain" comes from. The burn occurs in the muscle while it's being worked and often comes with fatigue and progressive weakness. It occurs during exercise, not at the start of exercise. It gets worse when pushing the endurance of the muscle (i.e. doing more reps). The burn often follows with a feeling of fullness in the muscle called "*the Pump*".
If you feel the burn and push through it with improper technique or "cheating" you can put yourself at risk for injury. As you train more, you will gain an appreciation for how much of the burn is tolerable without causing excessive strain or soreness the next day. The burn isn't necessary to make progress, but it is something that needs to be felt to shock the muscle into more rapidly adapting to training.

Sharp Pain

First of all, any sharp pain that comes suddenly during exercise, especially accompanied by a pop, crack, or snapping sensation, may indicate a significant injury. If you are lifting a weight and you feel a sharp pain that persists after you put the weight down stop exercising and seek medical attention from your athletic trainer, physical therapist, or physician. Same goes for other movements such as running, jumping, or twisting. Some injuries will be obvious as they can be incapacitating, cause a deformity, or have immediate swelling. If something swells up quickly after an injury this often represents bleeding from a tear or break in an anatomic structure such as a tendon, ligament, muscle, or bone. These injuries may even bruise within 24 hours.

Other sharp, shooting, or burning pain can be related to nerve problems. Pinched nerves in places like the neck, low back, elbow, or wrist can result in sharp pain that radiates across the extremity involved. Often this pain may present with numbness or tingling sensations and, in advanced stages, weakness or atrophy of a muscle group. You should always have these persistent nerve symptoms evaluated by a doctor.

Joint Pain and Swelling

If you have persistent pain and swelling around a joint this is more likely to be an injury. Most muscle bellies end before reaching a joint leaving ligaments, tendons, bursa, bone, and cartilage as the more likely sources of joint pain. Thus, persistent joint pain may represent tendonitis or tendon tear, bursitis, arthritis or cartilage injury, fracture, and even ligament injury or sprain. It is really not good to work through any joint related pain, unless confirmed by your physician as being OK. As we age many of us end up with mild and even advancing degenerative joint disease. In this case, one might need to work through a little bit of pain to keep the joint more supple and flexible, knowing that the intensity will need to be modified.

Disabling Pain

Pain that results in significant weakness or disability should always be evaluated. Certainly, DOMS can make one stiff and after a heavy training day perhaps a little weak, but this shouldn't be so weak that you have difficulty performing activities of daily living. Limping, inability to carry otherwise thought to be light objects, persistent low back/neck pain and/or numbness or tingling in the extremities, painful clicking, catching, locking, or instability of a joint all require medical attention. Beyond these musculoskeletal complaints, persistent fatigue, headaches, difficulty concentrating, fevers, chills, night sweats, unexplained weight loss or gain, palpitations, light-headedness, chest pain,

Anatomic Definitions:

Muscle:	Tissue that provides strength by contraction that moves joints.
Bone:	Load bearing structures containing calcium and phosphate that become stronger under stress. They also produce blood cells.
Tendons:	Thick bands of collagen that connect muscles to bone.
Ligaments:	Strong bands of collagen that connect one bone to another at joints.
Cartilage:	Layers of smooth lubricated tissue at the ends of bones that allow smooth motion of joints. Disruptions in the smooth gliding surfaces occurs in arthritis.
Bursa:	Small sacks of fluid that allow tendons to glide past bone or skin.

shortness of breath, bowel or bladder problems, or vision or hearing changes should all prompt a visit to a physician.

When in Texas, Don't Go Looking For Zebras

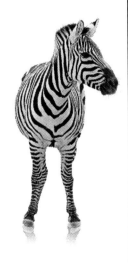

In medicine, we call rare conditions "Zebra's". When you are in Texas you are much more likely to find a horse than a Zebra (unless you're at the zoo). If you have a specific genetic predisposition to a rare disease because it's in your family, like being in the zoo, it may be more likely to find a Zebra in YOU. If this is not your case, common conditions are just more common. Duh! It is easy to go to the internet with a specific symptom and come up with all sorts of diagnoses that scare you into thinking that you need surgery or that you're going to die. I can't say that I haven't seen a rare cancer in a patient with knee pain. Nevertheless, avoid the anxiety produced by self-diagnosis and discuss any questions or concerns that you might have with your physician.

Masking the Pain – Why Anti-inflammatories Are Bad

One of the driving forces for the development of *The G.A.I.N. Plan* is the lack of guidance as to knowing when you have adequately recovered from an exercise training session. Overtraining or over-use is the root of most evil seen in my sports medicine practice. Tendinitis, stress fractures, bursitis, and arthritis are often due to excessive stress with inadequate recovery. I see this in my dancers and gymnasts who dance for 4 or 5 hours after school every day. They have an energy deficits leading to catabolism of muscle. Since they are training all day they never see the sun to get their vitamin D. All together this is a recipe for injury. Recovery should involve variations in training intensity and density, restful sleep, addressing daily stressors, and proper nutrition.

If a joint, tendon, or muscle group is giving you pain, it shouldn't be ignored or masked by anti-inflammatory medications. In fact, anti-inflammatory medications such as the NSAIDs (non-steroidal anti-inflammatory drugs) can perpetuate tendinitis and arthritis leading to more problems than good. Let's examine why.

Please Note: Abuse of NSAIDs leads to kidney disease, high-blood pressure, GI tract ulcers, and is number 1 cause of death from bleeding ulcers.

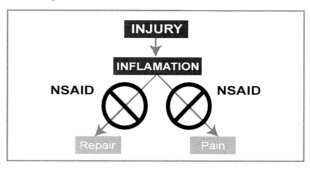

Inflammation is a process in your body which plays a huge role in tissue healing. Inflammatory white blood cells called neutrophils are attracted to sites of injury. When they arrive they release factors and attract other white cells called macrophages. Macrophages are big bulldozers that help to remove the bad tissue and initiate production of new tissue. They do this by releasing growth factors and chemicals, some of which are "pro-inflammatory". These lead to pain, increased blood flow, and swelling while others stimulate the formation of new tissues. The inflammatory cascade produces pain alerting you to the fact that tissue is being repaired and you need make some changes.

In addition to the growth factors, there are inflammatory mediators called "prostaglandins" that have the ability to stimulate the cells that are repairing the tissues in addition to causing pain. The non-steroidal anti-inflammatory drugs like ibuprofen or naproxen block the formation of prostaglandins. Thus, taking an NSAID masks the pain and allows you to workout with damaged and potentially unrepaired tissue. Now the tissue gets stressed by another workout and you end up in more pain when the NSAID wears off. Then you'll have a tendency to take more medication. Before too long you end up taking the medicine around the clock and continue to stress the tissue with inadequate time or stimulus for recovery. The end result is tissue damage that becomes irreparable and eventually scarred. Scar tissue will be weaker and less resilient than the original tissues.

In addition to obesity, NSAIDs may be contributing to the high rate of degenerative osteoarthritis in this country. Cartilage that cushions the bones at your joints can be damaged by injury or overuse and this damage can perpetuate into painful arthritis. Cartilage is a tissue with very little healing potential. When someone finds a way to reliably replace damaged cartilage they will likely get the Nobel Prize in medicine. Inhibiting the healing mediators of repair including prostaglandins can only lead to a decrease in tissue repair. In addition to the false sense of relief and early return to activity leads to further cartilage damage and delayed healing.

In cases of inflammatory arthritis, like rheumatoid arthritis, NSAIDs become necessary to calm down an overzealous inflammatory cascade. Without a diagnosis of inflammatory arthritis you should avoid regular NSAID use.

Besides joint cartilage, tendons can have mechanical strain from a stressful workout and end up scarring without normal tissue repair because of NSAID inhibition of reparative prostaglandins. Thus, the tendons become weaker and more susceptible to rupture. If you are using NSAIDs to calm down tendinitis, you should be modifying your activity to avoid disaster.

NSAIDs Block Muscle Growth!

The moral of the NSAID story is that pain is the body trying to tell you that something is wrong. Pain should be a guide to say that you have injured something or that you are overtraining. It needs to be a signal to you to work on helping your body actively recover with techniques presented here in *The G.A.I.N. Plan*. If you are on NSAIDs to relieve pain, make sure they are out of your system before your next workout, so that your pain is not masked. Besides, evidence suggests that NSAIDs may actually inhibit your muscles from growing in response to exercise. Why waste your hard training? We will examine this concept more in the next section.

Overcoming Injury

"It is defeat that turns bone to flint; it is defeat that turns gristle to muscle; it is defeat that makes men invincible." – Henry Ward Beecher

Beyond injury avoidance, it is important to be aware of ways to continue your progress in the unfortunate event of an injury. Of course, I will preface this section with the statement, "You should consult your treating physician before you embark on any of *The G.A.I.N. Plan* recommendations." In essence, I would like you to be able to take the suggestions I make in this book to your physician to show that you are informed and aware of alternatives. By the way, lawyers did not prompt me to make this statement; I truly believe you and your personal doctor need to be team players. For instance, nutritional supplementation may be beneficial to your recovery from surgery. As a physician on the GNC Medical Advisory Board, I have a unique perspective on supplement use around surgery. If you share some of these concepts with your physician, they may be enlightened and agreeable to change.

One of the most difficult challenges presented to a *G.A.I.N. Planner* is the unexpected injury. Injuries are going to happen in any sport done with competitive intensity. Some can be prevented with training techniques that prepare you for your sport. For instance, there are a number of exercises that can be done to help prevent non-contact ligament injuries in the knee (like ACL tear). Balance training, core exercises, agility training, and proprioceptive exercises can all facilitate performance while boosting injury avoidance. Avoiding extreme fatigue during risky movements like Olympic lifts, cutting sports, or jumping is very important when trying to avoid injury. However, when injuries occur it is important to realize that in most situations an injury presents a unique opportunity to take a step back, analyze your training, and work on visualization and weaknesses.

There are many conditions that can be caused by tight muscles, tendons, and joints. A tight muscle can lead to strain or tearing of the muscle during a ballistic activity. Also, a tight muscle causes excess tension on its tendon which attaches it to bone. Extra tension on tendons causes strain on the bone which causes tendinitis and bone spur formation. The constant excessive tension can lead to inflammation and micro-tearing of the tendon (tendonitis) which if left unchecked can lead to a ruptured tendon needing surgical repair! (See Stretching)

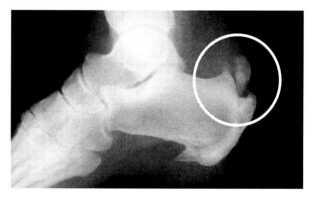

When you have inflammation around your joints and tendons it is important to give the affected body part "relative rest". Relative rest means that the stressful activity of that tendon needs to be cut back, but activity is not necessarily stopped altogether. For instance patellar tendonitis at the knee (Called "jumpers knee") needs avoidance of impact activity to calm down. The relative rest means that you would avoid jumping and running, but you would continue stretching and eccentric strengthening to rehab the tendon. It also means that you can train around the injury. This means avoiding the insulting activities, while working different exercises or body parts.

In dancers who have a stress fracture in their foot, relative rest may include doing barre exercises in the pool which off-loads your bodyweight. They may also do calisthenics while in a protective boot. This might include weight training without bearing weight on the affected foot, swimming, or a recumbent bike. Injuries in the upper or lower extremities often present a unique opportunity to focusing on strengthening the opposite end.

"Cross Education" to Keep Muscle!

Another principle is also under-utilized by many athletes called "cross education". Although the mechanisms aren't well known, when your brain sends signals to your arms or legs during an activity it is a bit of a mixed signal. Even if you aren't moving one of your arms or legs (i.e. in a cast or sling) the brain sends nerve signals to both sides. These nerve signals cause a release of growth factors at the muscle that help prevent atrophy from disuse of the extremity. This is a powerful technique that I have employed in every injury that I've had. Thus, I recommend that when one side is injured, strength training for the opposite side should not be neglected. I used this technique with sports supplements to limit atrophy in my bicep after repair.

Osteoarthritis

Over time, the build-up of years of training can lead to arthritis in joints, especially from impact sports. This is called degenerative joint disease or "osteo"arthritis (OA). OA is a progressive process; the speed at which the damage accumulates is different for each person and joint. The progression can be affected by genetic, biological, or biomechanical factors. It causes stiffness, swelling, achy to sharp pain, deformity and weakness.

It is well known that exercise, especially weight control, is beneficial to osteoarthritic joints. However, high impact activities or extraordinary loading can exacerbate the condition. If you have OA you need to keep working out, but you may need to adjust your training volume and intensity to avoid flare ups and disability. Occasional NSAIDs like ibuprofen, anti-inflammatory fish oils, glucosamine sulfate, and other herbal joint formulas may help you get started but shouldn't be relied on to get through every day.

Nutrition contributes to limiting systemic inflammation and increases in body weight which increase the pain associated with OA. Diets rich in omega-3 fatty acids and antioxidants may help with the joint pain and inflammation from OA. If you have joint replacements or have had other types of surgery for OA you may need to adjust your training to increase the longevity of the implant.

The "A"ttitude pillar of *G.A.I.N.* has intricate connections to joint inflammation and pain. As we pointed out earlier (*The G.A.I.N. Plan Mentality*), the FDA recently approved use of the anti-depressant medication Cymbalta for treatment of OA pain. Psychological stressors are a major player in symptoms of chronic arthritis pain. Scientists at the University of Wisconsin-Madison recognized this link and explored use of meditation techniques to limit symptoms in chronic inflammatory conditions. They used a Mindfulness-Based Stress Reduction

(MBSR) intervention to test its efficacy in treating stress and inflammation. They subjected the participants to a social stress test and an inflammation causing topical irritant. Those who used the 8 week MBSR intervention had a reduction in the inflammatory response despite having the same cortisol response to stress as the control group. They suggest that this meditation technique reduces emotional reactivity to inflammation and may be more beneficial than simply applying well-being promoting activities like diet and exercise.

Exercise, healthy diet, and mindfulness techniques constitute the fountain of youth. When the regions with the healthiest and longest living people are examined they are found to have a healthy diet, are relatively active, and have close social networks. The diets are rich in omega-3 and polyunsaturated fatty acids, green vegetables, lean meats, and whole grains. These populations are active in working outdoors, walking more than driving, and active hobbies. They also have close family ties and pay more attention to spiritual aspects of life. *The G.A.I.N. Plan* embraces these communities and gives you guidance in implementing this type lifestyle.

Having Surgery?

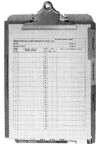

Even those who train cautiously and take good care of their body may end up in the office of a surgeon. Whether you have a meniscal tear in your knee, a tendon tear in your shoulder, or a hernia in your abdomen, surgery always presents an unplanned challenge to the athlete. As a high school athlete I had the dubious pleasure of experiencing both meniscal surgery on my knee and having hernia surgery in one year. Add on an appendectomy and a bicep

tendon repair during my residency, I have gained
an appreciation for how difficult it is to be an
athlete held back by such an injury.

*"There are no minor surgeries only minor
surgeons."* — Dr. Bill Hamilton

As an orthopaedic surgeon who has had multiple
surgeries, I have an appreciation not only for
what it takes to get a patient back to the playing
field, but also how anxious one can become
during the recovery process. The key to getting
through surgery is patience and persistence.
You must be patient with the healing process. As
much as patients and surgeons try to speed up
the healing process, there are some things that
just take time to heal. For instance, as a general
rule, we in orthopaedics say that it takes tendons
and ligaments approximately 6 weeks to heal
after injury or repair. Depending on the strength
of surgical repair, you may be able to rehab faster
when the repair is strong or you may be required
to hold back in tenuous repairs. When an injury
takes longer to recover than expected it is very
easy to get discouraged.

It is very important that you keep your long-
term goals in mind and keep a positive mental
attitude. This takes persistence by you, your
trainers, and your coaches. It is rare to have an
injury that completely disables you from being
able to train. It is very easy for a conservative
surgeon to say you are not allowed back in the
gym at "at all" until you have healed. This is
a surgeon who doesn't understand you as an
athlete. It is possible that there is a real reason
for this, but you may want to consider a second
opinion if during your preoperative evaluation

the surgeon says you will be unable to do any training over the next 3 months. Patients with lower extremity injuries (i.e. knee surgery, Achilles surgery, hip surgery) can train their upper body and core and vice versa.

Once you have found a surgeon who you think understands you as an athlete (that is for elective surgery; emergency surgery may leave you no choice until after) it is very important that you follow your surgeon's advice. If they tell you that you can't put weight on your foot for 6 weeks, then use your crutches religiously; don't "test it out". When your surgeon tells you it is OK to begin an activity again, don't assume that you will be able to go back to the same level of performance the next day. The longer you have been away from your discipline the longer it will take to return to it.

When I suggest that a patient goes back to sport after any injury, I teach them to take 2 steps forward with expectations that there will always be one step back. If you are just beginning to walk again, you don't begin by jogging. Walking with full weight may even be too much. If you were on crutches, take your time with getting rid of them. For instance, if your surgeon says that you are ready to begin bearing full weight try walking around with some weight on the leg using both crutches for support. This may make you sore later or experience some reactive swelling. Consider the swelling or soreness to be the one step back. Give it a little bit of a break to let the swelling and soreness come down and then try again, maybe this time you do a little bit more. Eventually using this step-wise process you wean from two crutches, to one crutch, and then to none. The same principles can be applied to the upper extremity (i.e. shoulder or elbow) with regards to getting back to weight training or throwing. Just because your doctor says that your rotator cuff is healed, doesn't mean that you're ready to throw. You, your doctor, and your physical therapist should lay out a specific plan to get back to your sport. Keep in mind, however, that the plan may need to be adjusted based on your progress or obstacles along the way.

When it comes to recovery, everyone is different. Delays can happen; your tear was worse, your condition had been going on for longer, or your healing is slower. Regardless, just because the guy next to you at therapy seems to be progressing faster, this doesn't mean that your surgery was done poorly or you are failing. Focus on your own rehabilitation and what your body and surgeon are telling you. If you are having persistent pain or swelling you may be doing too much or you may have a problem with healing your repair. If there is any doubt in your mind, seek the opinion of your surgeon.

There are many ways that you or your surgeon may speed up your recovery. One often overlooked way to improve recovery is through proper nutrition and use of nutritional supplementation. There may also be ways that the supplements or medications that you are already taking may affect the healing process, and necessitate cessation prior to surgery or treatment.

Perioperative Nutrition

As an athlete I have always been aware of the importance of nutrition and nutritional supplementation in improving performance. As a surgeon I have applied that same awareness to my surgical cases. The nutritional status of a patient is a huge factor in recovery from surgery. Many different tissue types need to heal after even the simplest of orthopaedic surgeries; the incision, bone, blood vessels, tendons, ligaments, cartilage, and more.

There are numerous scientific studies that support attention to nutrition around the time of surgery. This is especially important in those undergoing elective surgeries like an ACL Reconstruction or Rotator cuff repair, as you can proactively improve your diet to maximize your outcomes. Chances are that if you are reading this you are already trying to change your diet and life-style in away conducive to successful surgery.

In addition to a healthy balanced diet rich in low-fat proteins and veggies, I often make the following recommendations for perioperative nutrition:

1.   HAVE A CARBOHYDRATE LOAD THE NIGHT BEFORE:

     Most surgeries require at least a 6 hour fast prior to anesthesia. Usually, this is to avoid any aspiration of stomach contents during the anesthesia induction. In some cases you are told to have nothing to eat or drink after midnight the night before. Well, this can be pretty tolerable if you are the first case in the surgeon's day starting at 7am. However, delays happen all the time in the operating room. If you are the 3rd or 4th case, chances are you may be waiting 12-16 hours from your last meal before having surgery. As a result you are essentially going into the surgery malnourished.

Research shows that a carbohydrate rich meal prior to surgery can help build up glycogen stores to resist such an overnigh fast. I would highly recommend eating your last meal as close to your bed time the night before as possible. Have complex carbohydrates (75-100g, yams, rice, potatoes), a healthy protein (Fish, chicken breast, lean beef, etc), and veggies. Avoid high fat and fried foods the night before Saturated fat and omega-6 rich fats may increase the inflammation post-operatively Consider having and omega-3 rich food like salmon to reduce your inflammation and pain post-operatively.

2. TAKE YOUR MULTIVITAMIN:

    Although some surgeons say to stop your multivitamin prior to surgery for fear that you are taking a supplement that thins your blood, I believe that a regular strength multivitamin with minerals is safe to have up to the day of most surgeries. The essential vitamins and minerals are helpful for wound healing and are critical antioxidants in time of stress. I recommend paying particular attention to taking your multivitamin regularly up to 3 weeks before surgery and 6 weeks thereafter.

3. TAKE 500MG VITAMIN C:

    Vitamin C has been shown to limit the incidence of a complication that can occur with all surgeries. Complex regional pain syndrome (CRPS) is a condition that can make even the best surgery go bad. We do not know what the exact cause of CRPS is but it is obviously complex. We do know that after sustaining a wrist fracture, taking 500mg of Vitamin C for the first 6 weeks helps prevent the formation of CRPS which is relatively common in this condition. It is believed that the antioxidant effect of the Vitamin C plays a role. Vitamin C is also an important nutrient in collagen formation and thus wound, tendon, ligament, and bone healing.

4. CONSIDER A PROTEIN SUPPLEMENT:

   I always recommend whey protein shakes or at least any additional protein that one can take in the pre and post-operative period. Some patients may be a little malnourished going into surgery and require a few weeks of supplemental protein for maximizing nutritional markers, Vegetarians can use soy protein supplements. Going through surgery can be as stressful as running a marathon. You need to fuel recovery just as you would a tough workout.

5. HAVE A FOOD SUPPLEMENT/RTD AVAILABLE FOR FIRST DAY AFTER SURGERY:

   It is always a good idea to have a meal replacement protein drink or "ready-to-drink" protein available for the day of surgery. Try something in the week before surgery so that you know you like the taste and that it is appealing to you. You may be nauseated after surgery either from the anesthesia or from the pain medicines you might take afterwards. The pain may even make sitting up for a full meal difficult or uncomfortable. If you have a protein shake that you can sip on you can be certain to get critical nutrients needed for healing. Also, by getting some nutrition you will help reduce your stress hormone levels. I recommend to my patients that they continue to use the shakes until they feel like they have gotten back into their normal healthy dietary habits.

6.   CALCIUM AND VITAMIN D:

Calcium and Vitamin D are clearly important in healing of bone. If you are having surgery involving bone healing (fracture repair, osteotomy, fusion surgery) it is important that you have your vitamin D levels checked pre-operatively. If you are deficient your physician may recommend supplementation. I have had patients who presented to me with bones that just won't heal only to discover vitamin D deficiency. After supplementation with vitamin D and use of a bone stimulator, many of these patients can avoid revision surgery and go on to solid bone healing. The typical dose of vitamin D is 400iu twice per day. However, I am a proponent of up to 1000iu twice per day and more in those who are resistant to restoration of blood levels. Calcium is taken at a dose of 500mg twice per day.

7.   GLUCOSAMINE SULFATE:

Glucosamine is a critical component of your articular cartilage. This is the lining of your joints at the ends of your bones that provides smooth gliding surfaces for the joint. When damaged this causes mechanical clicking, catching, and locking in the joint along with swelling and pain. Badly damaged cartilage leads to degenerative arthritis. In randomized, placebo controlled studies; glucosamine sulfate (not glucosamine hydrochloride) has demonstrated beneficial effects for cartilage damage and joint pain. The articular cartilage has a relatively high amount of sulfate. I believe that the sulfate version of glucosamine is more beneficial because of the affinity for sulfate to the joint. Some surgeons may not want you to take glucosamine sulfate if you are on a blood thinner for its theoretical risk of increasing bleeding. I recommend any of my cartilage repair patients to use 500mg of glucosamine sulfate three times per day during their post-op rehabilitation. In addition, fish oil supplements help with reducing joint inflammation and pain and are thus good additions to the glucosamine. Fish oil use may also need to be delayed until the risk of bleeding subsides. As with glucosamine this is a topic of scientific discussion. When it comes to any adjustments in your lifestyle or diet, you should discuss this with your surgeon. Some surgeons are not as "in-tune" with nutrition and supplementation around surgery. If your surgeon doesn't seem to hold particular interest in these things you could certainly consult with a nutritionist.

Biological Ways to Improve Recovery

There are many new biological methods being developed and marketed for the improvement of the healing process. This has become big business in recent years. Unfortunately, the science of these methods is in its infancy and is still quite controversial. Most of the benefit of these methods has been validated in the laboratory, but lacks clinical evidence to recommend them universally in humans. Presented here are a few of those treatment methods. As an orthopaedic surgeon I am an advocate of biological healing techniques. The evidence is strong enough for improvement in pain control, wound healing, and tissue healing during Achilles tendon surgery and cartilage surgery that I use Stem cells or Platelet-rich Plasma regularly.

Stem Cells: Your surgeon may harvest stem cells from your pelvic bone or fat tissue in order to improve healing of bone, tendons, or ligaments. Stem cells are cells that have the ability to become almost any type of tissue and grow and develop based on the environment in which they are placed.

Growth Factors: These are proteins that act as signaling molecules between cells. They act to stimulate the growth and differentiation of cells. For instance, a growth factor called bone morphogenic protein "BMP" stimulates stem cells to become bone cells. BMPs made in the laboratory can be applied to the site of a surgery or injury to stimulate the healing of the tissue of interest.

Platelet-Rich Plasma (PRP): Platelets are tiny little cell like structures that are found in high numbers in your blood. They play a critical role in forming a clot at the site of a wound by clumping together. They contain many compounds, including growth factors that help heal whatever wound they form a clot in. PRP is made using peripheral blood (from a blood draw at your arm) that is spun down in a centrifuge to separate out the "platelet-rich" portion of the blood plasma. This concentrated collection of platelets can be applied to the site of an injury or surgery and presumably improves the healing process by delivering more stimulatory growth factors.

For Men Only?

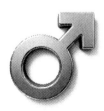

Testosterone Physiology: Testosterone is a steroid hormone made from cholesterol in the testes and is released in a circadian fashion. The term "circadian" refers to the daily rise and fall of testosterone with the highest levels generally occurring in the morning and lowest at bedtime; hence morning erections. This must be kept in mind when assessing your own testosterone with blood work. Be consistent in the time at which you have your levels drawn in a lab. Moreover, if you notice that your morning erections are getting soft or not at all, get your morning testosterone levels checked as you are likely deficient.

Testosterone production and release is controlled by the hypothalamus. The hypothalamus has intricate connections to higher brain functions which make it sensitive to environmental stress and stimuli. Many events in your world can effect testosterone production such as driving a fast car, seeing a sexy woman, jumping out of a plane, or squatting 400lbs. The hypothalamus releases luteinizing hormone-releasing hormone (LHRH) which acts directly on the pituitary gland to stimulate release of luteinizing hormone (LH). LH then reaches the testes where it stimulates testosterone production and release.

Testosterone is carried through the blood on proteins. In particular, the protein sex hormone-binding globulin (SHBG) carries up to 60% of your testosterone. The rest is bound to serum albumin and a small fraction, usually around 2% is free or unbound. The "free" fraction is the most active form of the hormone. The free testosterone interacts with receptors inside your cells that act directly on DNA to make specific proteins to promote its agenda. Testosterone can also act through derivatives dihydrotestosterone (DHT) made by 5α-reductase and estrogen made by aromatase.

Testosterone's agenda is to make you a man. Unless you are a woman, then testosterone helps with libido, bone density, and lean muscle mass. Testosterone plays a vital role in your development from the point of conception and well into old age. Your development of male sexual characteristics is a result testosterone's anabolic (muscle building) and androgenic (body hair, sex drive, etc) activity rising during critical phases in development like puberty. Aging beyond 35-40 years is associated with a 1-3% decline per year in circulating testosterone concentration in men.

Muscular Development and Fat

When testosterone acts on a muscle cell it has
multiple actions that increase muscle protein
content. First, it stimulates the uptake of
amino acids into muscle cells and promotes
the synthesis of muscle proteins. Second,
testosterone has anti-catabolic properties,
which is to say that it prevents the breakdown of
muscle. It does this by limiting muscle glycogen
breakdown and blocking the effect of the
hormone cortisol. Cortisol is released as a result
of external environmental stress which leads
to a need for the mobilization of carbohydrates
and consumption of muscle proteins for vital
functions; it is the quintessential catabolic
hormone.

Free testosterone levels correlate well with
muscle strength, bone mineral density, and
lower levels of body fat in elderly men. Obesity
is associated with physiological changes in
circulating sex steroid levels. Obese men have
more aromatase activity which is an enzyme that
converts testosterone to estrogens in peripheral
tissues such as fat. Circulating levels of
testosterone lower than 230ng/dL are associated
with severe impairments in body composition
and glucose metabolism. Many correlations
can be made between low testosterone and the
"metabolic syndrome" of insulin resistance,
abnormal cholesterol, high blood pressure, and
abdominal obesity.

Thus, maintaining and improving testosterone
levels has been a topic of great interest to doctors
and athletes alike ever since its discovery. As
levels of testosterone drop with age men in

their 40s to 50s may relate to feelings of fatigue, depression, loss of vitality, decreased libido, and loss of strength and muscle mass. Some think it really isn't so much where your testosterone levels are at, but more where they are going. As we said earlier there is quite a significant variation in testosterone levels throughout the day so it takes relatively large drops or rises to break a threshold that results in symptoms or improvements muscle, respectively.

When we examine rises and falls in testosterone as a result of exercise or nutritional supplements we must keep this threshold in mind. Small changes in testosterone throughout the day are unlikely to have a large impact on muscle growth and recovery. Anyone who has taken testosterone injections will tell you that unless you're taking 200 mg or more per week you are not going to get a significant bodybuilding response. This type of dosing can bring someone easily from a level of 400 to 1200 or a 300% rise in your levels. So we must be cautious when we look at studies that raise measured testosterone by 20 or even 40% and jump to conclusions that this will lead to significant body composition changes. In fact, the best way to experience a rise in testosterone *and* experience body composition changes is to raise your levels with proper exercise and nutrition.

Exercise, Rest and Testosterone Levels

As we discussed, testosterone builds muscle and so does exercise. There is a definite correlation between elevated testosterone and muscle growth. Weight training stimulates muscle strength and hypertrophy (growth) which is in part due to increases in testosterone.

*HIIT
Boosts
Testosterone!*

Most bodybuilders know that there is a constant battle in the body between catabolic cortisol and anabolic testosterone. Some believe that doing concurrent strength training with aerobic conditioning puts these hormones in competition with one another. Plenty of research shows that overtraining or long distance endurance training results in significant elevations is cortisol and these are sustained elevations over weeks of training. Weight training can cause a cortisol stress response but the body quickly adapts and the levels drop for the same intensity of training as testosterone elevates or stays the same. The cortisol response may be even more pronounced in women. However, research supports that strength training can restore the anabolic balance to moderate endurance training. Better yet, high intensity interval endurance training supports healthy testosterone increases by 60 to 97%. Evidence also confirms that changes in testosterone or cortisol concentrations can support neuromuscular performance through various short-term mechanisms (e.g. second messengers, lipid/protein pathways, neuronal activity, behavior, cognition, motor-system function, muscle properties and energy metabolism).

Loebel and Kraemer explained the testosterone response to exercise succinctly . There are many variables to weight training programs, and they can affect the endocrine response to that training. Varying the exercises, order of exercise, sets, rest between sets, reps and weight can all affect testosterone levels. Kraemer showed that training for muscle growth with 10 rep maximums for multiple exercises with 1 min rests produced a greater magnitude of increase in testosterone than a 5 rep maximum load with 3 min rest. Overall the testosterone response post-exercise is fairly consistent with many variations in volume and intensity of weight training for mass. However, looking at the numbers closely we are talking about a rise in levels of testosterone on a magnitude of 15-20% on average or maximally 90-100% with HIIT. Although this is better than a drop seen with many forms of lengthy endurance exercise, this is very small when you consider the effects of supplemental testosterone which can increase levels by 300 to 500% from baseline. Nonetheless, even short-term rises above baseline have beneficial effects on exercise physiology as supported by literature.

Most importantly and left for last, rest and recovery are of great importance in maintaining healthy testosterone levels. Overtraining, regardless of the type of exercise performed increases cortisol levels and depresses testosterone levels. Many of the recuperative effects controlled by anabolic hormones are affected by sleep. Hormones such as testosterone and growth hormone rise after a good night of sleep. Remember, what you do outside the gym is often as important as or more important than what you do inside the gym. That's why we call it a bodybuilding *lifestyle*.

Nutrition, Supplements, and Testosterone Levels

There are many studies, old and new, that support the effects that diet can have on endocrine responses in humans and animals. On the extremes, such as a vegetarian diet or very low calorie diets, we know that these can be detrimental to testosterone levels. High fiber and low cholesterol or diets severely restricted in fat reduce the availability of the precursors of testosterone synthesis and can potentially decrease testosterone levels. Additionally, diets with protein providing more than 40% of calories vs. 15% protein calories have higher testosterone levels in some studies but the effects of macronutrient composition on endocrine function is inconsistent and controversial.

There are many different herbs and plant derived compounds that can affect your testosterone levels, but most of the research is quite superficial, inconsistent and heavily biased by manufacturers. That being said there are a few compounds that are worth noting as they have some relatively stronger research backing. Also I must note that even though these compounds have been shown to have modest effects on testosterone levels (mostly in animals), often this has not been correlated to improved physiques or strength.

TRIBULUS TERRESTRIS (TT) is a flowering plant found in the temperate and tropical regions of Southern Asia, Africa, and Australia. It has long been described as a treatment for male sexual dysfunction and was popularized by research from a Bulgarian pharmaceutical company with Tribestan suggesting it could increase testosterone. However, these studies aren't available for scrutiny. Multiple studies have been performed in rodents and have demonstrated an increase in testosterone levels with TT feeding. Conversely human trials of isolated TT extract supplementation have failed to show consistent rises in testosterone and/or accretion of lean body mass without having significant industry bias.

D-ASPARTIC ACID (DAA) is an amino acid found concentrated in the testes, hypothalamus, and pituitary. Italian scientists published a study in 2009 which brought DAA to the forefront in testosterone boosters. Feeding DAA to rats is capable of eliciting the release of the gonadotropin-releasing hormone (GnRH) from the hypothalamus, the luteinizing hormone (LH) and the growth hormone (GH) from the pituitary gland, and testosterone from the testes. Furthermore, supplementing humans with 12 days of 3.12g of DAA resulted in nearly a 30% increase in serum testosterone levels. The "however" is that DAA can accumulate in tissues and it is not clear how safe this is so I would recommend limiting the dose to 1g per day for a maximum of 8 weeks until further testing can be done.

ASTAXANTHIN + SAW PALMETTO is an herbal combination that in-vitro studies demonstrated a significantly greater inhibition of the enzyme 5α reductase (converts T to DHT) and aromatase (converts T to E). This herbal combination produced significant increases in serum testosterone levels up to 60% while decreasing estrogen and DHT. A dose of 800 and 2000mg were shown to equally raise testosterone levels, while 2000mg further increased the drop in estrogen. *Bias Alert:* the study was funded by the company that made the product.

FENUGREEK, TRIGONELLA FOENUM GRAECUM, commonly used as a spice in Middle Eastern countries and widely used in south Asia and Europe, are known to have anti-diabetic properties and an ability to boost testosterone levels. Interestingly it contains an unusual amino acid 4-hydroxyisoleucine, so far found only in fenugreek, which has anti-diabetic properties of enhancing insulin secretion under hyperglycaemic conditions, and increasing insulin sensitivity. Its ability to raise testosterone levels and improve insulin action explains its ability to produce an anabolic effect in humans and rats. In addition to doubling testosterone levels, Fenugreek has even been shown at a dose of 500mg to significantly impact both upper- and lower-body strength and body composition in comparison to placebo in a double blind controlled trial. Despite some good research, further evaluation of Fenugreek extract in resistance-trained males showed only a significant decrease in DHT levels and without a boost in testosterone.

MACUNA PRURIENS & WITHANIA SOMNIFERA are two other herbals are supported by human clinical studies to increase testosterone both at a dose of 5g/d: . These can significantly increase serum testosterone levels but in relatively high dosing and after 3 to 5 months of use. With such high dosing using these compounds may be a little impractical until exercise related studies show them to be beneficial.

BORON is a trace element nutrient that when supplied as a dietary supplement may increase the concentration of plasma steroid hormones. In a single blind cross-over trial, boron supplementation caused a significant increase in plasma 17-B estradiol (estrogens) concentration and there was a trend for plasma testosterone levels to be increased. The ratio of estradiol to testosterone increases significantly and rat studies support these findings.

Much of the research on boron supplementation and boosting of steroid hormone levels comes from a single lab, Naghii et al. in Iran. Their most recent study published in 2011 suggested that boron supplementation for a week at 10mg per day with breakfast increased free testosterone levels by ~28%. However, this time they found a reduction in estradiol concentration by 39%! The ratio of estrogen to testosterone was lower and in the opposite direction as the previous study. The reason for this discrepancy is really unexplainable.

I am always concerned when one lab produces the majority of positive results in humans with small participant numbers (n=10) and inconsistent results. If an independent lab shows a similar sustained rise in free testosterone in a larger study group with statistical significance, then I will believe in the potential of this compound. Remember more isn't better. Boron should not be taken above 20mg per day or it may become toxic.

In conclusion, testosterone plays a critical role in muscle anabolism and making you a healthy man. You should have your levels checked, especially if you are symptomatic of "Low T". If you plan to focus your diet or supplement routine on boosting testosterone levels don't go at it blindly. Just like watching your poundage's on the bench or your weight on the scale you should check your baseline morning testosterone level. If you take any of the above supplements, recheck your levels in a month or 2. If your levels go up and you see improvements in the gym go ahead and record your own statistical significance.

4. N: Nutrition

You Are What You Eat

I know it is an overused cliché, but it really has some truth. You are what you eat. Your food choices reflect your attitude, self-esteem, and desire to be healthy. The food you eat also affects all of the same including your appearance, energy level, stress, strength, well-being, and longevity. Our mouths are a gateway to our minds and bodies. What we say and what we put into our mouths affects our bodies, minds, and those around us. The food we eat obviously affects our bodies, but also affects our minds and those around us.

When you go out to eat with friends you have a unique opportunity to show off a lot about yourself. The food you choose from the menu reflects your goals, attitudes, and sense of well-being. When you choose fried, starchy, and calorie rich foods it reflects on your tendency to over-indulge and neglect your health. After reading this book you'll have a better understanding of healthy eating. The next time you go out, you will show off your knowledge and desire to live well by ordering foods with nutritional complexity. You will be able to explain to your friends why you're eating the way you are and teach them what you've learned in *The G.A.I.N. Plan*. You'll be a conversation starter and be the star of the table. Everyone is interested in eating right; eating badly is just a hard habit to break.

P.A.C.E. Your Foods

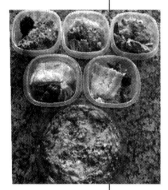

You can present your favorite meals and recipes on social media! Perform like a culinary master utilizing the concept of P.A.C.E. to show off your creations to your friends and the world on social media. You can continue to gain further motivation and stir up creativity from your Twitter followers and Facebook friends by posting your favorite recipes and pictures of your creations. Performing as a chef can be just as motivational as performing as an athlete. Some famous authors started this way before writing their recipe books. Share your recipes and see some of my favorites at yourgainplan.com.

Our diets are built from habit; which, of course, can be healthy or unhealthy. Many Americans are trapped in a cycle of unhealthy habits revolving around food. As we discussed early in the book, these habits can be deeply ingrained and in some cases can be considered an addiction. It may take some repetition and meditative introspection to overcome these bad habits.

Once you have read this section, you will have a better idea of what healthy eating is all about. I will discuss some common misconceptions about fats, proteins, and carbohydrates. I will go over the importance of balanced nutrition and timing of your meals. I will discuss how specific nutrients and deficiencies can affect your health, well-being, and performance. I will also discuss how nutritional supplementation can help you to reach your goals faster.

Energy Balance

Understanding nutrition requires an appreciation that every person's metabolism and activity level is different and thus you will have different nutritional needs than someone else. Your diet should not be a cookie cutter, eat one way, type of meal plan. Your nutrition is dynamic and must be well coordinated with your goals and your personal biometrics (i.e. energy expenditure). Whether you are looking to lose fat and gain muscle, improve your endurance, increase your strength, or even gain weight, your diet needs to be in-sync with your personal goals.

Undernourishment can be just as big a problem as over-nourishment. Clearly if you are over-nourished you will store the extra food and calories as fat; however, in order to gain muscle weight you need to eat enough calories and protein to fuel muscle growth. If your goal is to maintain or gain muscle, this really can't be done on a severely restricted diet. You can lose fat on this diet, but you will lose much muscle in the process. Under-nourishment, especially with extreme restriction is quite stressful on the body and leads to the problems associated with OTS as we discussed earlier in the book.

When you are training intensely you need plenty of food to remain *anabolic*. This means enough calories and protein to maintain muscle. If you restrict your caloric intake to excess, your body will go into *starvation mode*. In starvation mode your body tries to conserve energy and resources to protect your brain and other organs. Your basal metabolic rate slows down, you switch from a muscle growth mode to a muscle breakdown mode, fat stores limit the release of fat, and your body prepares for a famine by trying to store any extra calories that may pop in. *In essence, under-nourishment leads to a fatigued mind with a flabby body that becomes a sponge for calories.*

Carbohydrate, fat, and protein are converted into energy by working muscles to fuel day to day activities and exercise. The more active you are throughout the day and the more intense your training the more energy you expend. Thus it is important to consume calories proportionate to your energy expenditure. We have methods to calculate your daily energy expenditure based on statistical norms or based on direct measurements of activity. Biometric monitors can give you a fairly close estimate of your daily caloric expenditure based on activity level measured by accelerometer, heart rate, body temperature, and galvanic skin responses. If you don't have a monitor (I strongly recommend you try one) you can calculate your daily caloric expenditure and thus needs via a couple equations. In order to get a fairly accurate estimate of your energy needs you just need your height, weight, and age. If you want to get a more accurate measurement of your energy expenditure, measure your body fat percentage and plug it into the appropriate equation. By knowing your body fat percentage, you can determine how much lean mass you have; remember, muscle is "metabolic currency".

Basal Metabolic Rate (BMR) is a measure of the amount of energy in calories that your body burns if you are at complete rest for 24 hours. This is essentially the energy you burn if you were to just lay down on an empty stomach at neutral room temperature. This is the energy expended to keep vital organs functioning. It really is a nebulous number because we are never in this situation. BMR is affected by genetics, gender, age, weight, body surface area, body fat percentage, diet, temperature, hormones, the nervous system, and exercise. The simple act of eating food induces more caloric expenditure through "thermogenesis" and the muscle activity of eating.

Our warm-bloodedness is due to the fact that our bodies produce heat from chemical energy and muscle activity. Although we are insulated by white fat under our skin that stores energy, we are also born with a very special type of fat called "brown" fat (Brown Adipose Tissue or BAT) that generates heat. AT is very metabolically active tissue that generates a lot of heat from chemical energy. It is rich in proteins called "uncoupling" proteins (UCPs) that release large amounts of chemical energy as heat. The UCPs in BAT appear to be activated by the revved up, adrenalin infused sympathetic nervous system, cold environments, and certain foods. The "thermic effect of food" is food's ability to stimulate heat production in the body. Studies support that when meals are higher in protein and lower in fat they cause greater increases in thermic energy expenditure. Furthermore, supplements containing capsaicin appear to improve fat burning through the same thermic effect via activation of BAT. Studies also show that BAT energy expenditure increases by up to 10% if we just turn down the thermostat to ~65°F. Science is feverishly looking for more ways to turn on your BAT.

The **Harris-Benedict (H-B) Equation** can be used to calculate your BMR based on your height, weight, age, and sex. If you have calculated your body fat percentage you can use **the Katch-McArdle (K-M) Formula** to get a more accurate estimate of your BMR. By knowing how much lean body mass (proportional to the amount of muscle you have) you'll have a measure of your "metabolic currency". I highly recommend that you learn to use a skin-fold caliper as one of your objective measures of progress.

The more muscle you have the more energy your body burns at rest. This is why I find it so important that we focus on building and maintaining muscle. *K-M* represents your actual body composition and is not based on assumptions about how many calories an individual should consume. Also, since *K-M* formula includes a measurement of *actual* lean body mass it applies to both men and women, whereas the H-B equation assumes that a man has more lean body mass than a woman based on statistical norms.

It is important to note that this is all just an estimate. You will have to follow tour progress (BW, BF%, mirror, etc.) and adjust your energy balance accordingly.

Harris- Benedict Equation
Men:

BMR = 66.5 + (13.75 x weight in kg) + (5.0 x height in cm) − (6.75 x age in years)

Women:
BMR = 655.1 + (9.56 x weight in kg) +
(1.85 x height in cm) − (4.67 x age in years)

Katch-McArdle,Formula:
BMR = 370 + (21.6 X lean mass in kg)

Calculation for Lean Mass
BF% x total body weight= *total fat weight*
therefore:

Lean mass in kg = total body weight −
total fat weight

Once you have your BMR you need to consider
how active you are to get your total daily energy
expenditure. Again, an activity monitor can help
you to be more accurate with this measurement
otherwise we need to use standardized numbers.
The Katch-Mcardle Formula provides activity
factors that can be applied to either of the BMR
formulas above. Just multiply your BMR by
the Activity Factor and you will have a simple
estimate of the total calories you burn each day.

Activity Factors:
- *If you are Sedentary
  (little or no exercise)*:
  Calorie-Calculation = BMR X **1.2**

- *If you are Lightly Active
  (light exercise/sports 1-3 days/week)*:
  Calorie-Calculation = BMR X **1.375**

- *If you are Moderately Active
  (moderate exercise/sports 3-5 days/week)*:
  Calorie-Calculation = BMR X **1.55**

- *If you are Very Active
  (hard exercise/sports 6-7 days/week):*
  Calorie-Calculation = BMR X **1.725**

- *If you are Extra Active
  (very hard daily exercise/sports & physical
  job or 2X day training):*
  Calorie-Calculation = BMR X **1.9**

Now that you have a way to roughly determine your energy expenditure each day, you should write this number down so that you can understand how to adjust your diet to meet your energy needs. If you are trying to maintain your weight, you need to the minimum number of calories provided by these equations. It should be noted that in extremely muscular or extremely obese people these numbers may be way off. You also need to realize that these numbers are not going to match your expenditure every day. Some days it may be a low estimate, some days it may be high. At the end of the week you need to assess if you are losing weight or gaining weight and adjust your diet accordingly.

1lb of Fat = 3500 Calories

You can estimate body fat adjustments based on the assumption that a pound of fat is equivalent to ~3500 Calories. This is a very imprecise number, but it is close enough to an average that many nutritionists use it. To lose 1 lb of fat in a week, you need to burn or cut 500 calories/day from your diet below your needs. To avoid the starvation response, it is best to do this by burning 250 extra calories in the form of exercise, while limiting food intake by 250 calories. Very roughly, with regards to food intake, men should avoid going much lower than 1500 calories per day, while women should avoid going below 1200 calories per day. If a larger deficit is needed than 500 calories, this should be done through added exercise. Resistance exercise will give a muscle growth stimulus to counter balance the catabolism. As we will discuss, if the right nutrients are on board, the muscle loss will be minimized in larger energy deficits.

Primer on Macronutrients

Macronutrients are the fats, carbohydrates, and proteins that are our main sources of energy. The *micronutrients* are those nutrients that are consumed in small quantities such as in vitamins and minerals and are not considered an energy source. Of the three macronutrients there are only 2 that are absolutely essential in our diet.

Without certain fats we could not survive because there are essential fats that are bodies need but cannot make. The *essential fatty acids* include *alpha-linolenic acid* (an omega-3 fatty acid) and *linoleic acid* (an omega-6 fatty acid). Fats are found in our bodies as triglycerides. *Triglycerides* consist of 3 fatty acid chains attached to a glycerol molecule. They are stored in fat cells and carried in the blood. Fats are the most energy dense of the macronutrients providing 9 calories per gram.

There are also *essential amino acids* which are the building blocks of protein that our bodies can't synthesize from other nutrients. Without eating those amino acids, certain biological processes and tissues would fail or die. We can get all of the essential amino acids by eating "complete" proteins. There are forms of protein, such as many plant derived proteins, that are lacking in at least one essential amino acid and are thus considered "incomplete" proteins. Amino acids can be used as fuel and generate 4 calories per gram.

Conversely, there are *no essential carbohydrates* in our diet. Carbohydrates are composed of small units called *monosaccharides* which include glucose, fructose, and galactose. Monosaccharides and *disaccharides* (2 monosaccharides combined) like table sugar called sucrose (glucose + fructose) and lactose from dairy (glucose + galactose) are considered "simple sugars". *Polysaccharides* can be long chains of monosacchrides and are referred to as starches or *complex carbohydrates*. The polysaccharides that we can't digest or absorb are called *fiber*. One could argue that fiber is the essential only carbohydrate: see Pre-biotics.

Glucose is stored in muscle and the liver in a chain called *glycogen*, which is an easily accessible albeit small energy source for muscle. Carbohydrates also generate 4 calories per gram.

Our bodies have the ability to produce all the glucose it needs to maintain a functioning brain from the other macronutrients. For instance, the glycerol backbone released from the metabolism of fat can be used in a process called *gluconeogenesis* (production of glucose). As for the amino acids, all can be converted into substrates for gluconeogenesis except for leucine and lysine. When glycogen stores are depleted, in muscle during exertion and the liver during fasting, catabolism of muscle proteins to amino acids contributes the major source of carbon for maintenance of blood glucose levels.

The liver can also make *ketones* from fatty acids to fuel the heart and brain in times of low carbohydrate. A very low carbohydrate diet can lead to fat conversion to ketones which accumulate in the blood in a process called "Ketosis". Some believe that this "ketogenic diet' burns fat faster and more efficiently. There is data to support these assertions. However, these diets can be quite challenging.

The Skinny on Fats

In the 1980's all fats were vilified. Do you remember all the "fat-free" this and that commercials? The fat-free craze led to manufacturers replacing fat with sugars for palatability. As a result, we have become more obese and insulin resistant than ever before. In this section, I will review how certain fats are not only essential to your health but are able to boost your performance in the gym.

The 80s No Fat Fad

One of the biggest public policy and marketing mistakes of the food industry and government regulation of nutrition was the "No Fat Fad" in the late 1980s. As was mentioned in the myth section, Dr. Ancel Keys perpetuated a myth of toxic fat based on flawed science. Furthermore, media and the manufacturing industry over-generalized saturated fats to mean all fats are bad. Thus, the "no fat" food barrage ensued.

Saturated fats and thus all fats were deemed to be the enemy of cardiovascular health and longevity. As a result, industry ran with the hype and started producing low or no fat food. Fat provides a significant amount of palatability to a food. In order to restore food palatability, industry replaced fats with sugars.

At that point, the evils of sugar weren't on the radar. As a result the average intake of refined sugars such as high fructose corn syrup increased significantly. From what you have already learned in this book about the evils of sugar, you can understand the consequences of such a disaster of marketing and policy. Companies like Archer Daniels Midland (ADM) made a fortune on the boost in corn syrup demand. In fact, ADM's sales have more than tripled in the last 10 years.

Become a proponent of sugar avoidance. Help those around you to recognize that sugars, syrups, and juices equate to toxins. These sugars lead to diabetes, metabolic syndrome, obesity, cancer, and heart disease. After reading The G.A.I.N. Plan, *share what you have learned with everyone around you. Make a difference in your world.*

There are "essential" fatty acids and amino acids that we can't live without eating because our bodies can't make them. To suggest that we should live fat-free is an over simplification of the fact that most Americans need to consume less calories no matter which way they come. Since fats are calorie rich with 9 calories per gram vs. 4 calories per gram for protein and carbohydrate, they are often limited first by dieters. However, limiting sugar and carbohydrates should be their focus, while consuming healthier fats like omega-3 fish oils and monounsaturated fats from nuts over saturated animal fats.

In general, fats improve the digestion of your food. Fats delay emptying of food from your stomach just like bulky fiber does. Fattier foods sit in your stomach longer and are better digested. Additionally, by slowing the emptying of food from the stomach, sugars consumed in the meal reach your blood slower. In doing so, fats effectively reduce the glycemic index of a meal. Fats reduce the rapid rise in blood sugar that leads to insulin spikes to which your body becomes resistant as in type II diabetes. Further, certain fats (LC-PUFAs; see below) have greater ability to reduce appetite than others.

In addition to the digestive properties of fats, all fats are not created equal in their effects on your body. Fats aren't just a source of calories and insulation. Fats are essential for the health of your nerves, your skin, your muscles, your brain, your heart and more. Fats also make up the membranes of all of your cells and different fats have various effects on the fluidity of those membranes. Your cells make inflammatory mediators like prostaglandins from the fats in your cell membranes; various fats forming various mediators.

Fats are made of a glycerol backbone and chains of "fatty acids". Fatty acids are energy rich carbon chains that have many hydrogen atoms attached. When every carbon is full of hydrogen atoms a fat is considered "saturated". This is energy rich fat that solidifies at room temperature like lard.

The "unsaturated" fatty acids are oilier and have hydrogen's missing at various locations which impart in the fatty acid different biological and physical properties. When there are multiple carbon pairs missing hydrogen's in a fatty acid (this forms a carbon to carbon double bond C=C) we call the fatty acid a polyunsaturated fatty acid (PUFA). When the double bond (C=C) is at the third carbon atom from the end of the carbon chain the PUFA is called an Omega-3. Similarly, there are omega-6 and 9's with the last double bond at the 6th and 9th carbon from the end of the chain. When the fatty acid only has one C=C, it is called a mono-unsaturated fatty acid (MUFA).

The essential fatty acids that you can't live without are PUFA's including *a-linolenic acid* (ALA; an omega-3 short chain PUFA) and *linoleic* acid (an omega-6 short chain PUFA). These essential fatty acids are the foundation for the formation of long chain polyunsaturated fatty acids or "LC-PUFA's". That being said, LC-PUFA's are not essential if the short chain PUFA's are available.

The short chain PUFA's can be elongated to the LC-PUFA's in the body but microalgae in the ocean are much more adept at doing this than humans. The omega-3 LC-PUFA's which are much easier to get from fish that eat tons of algae are the 20 carbon *eicosapentaenoic acid* (EPA) and the even longer 22 carbon *docosahexaenoic acid* (DHA). Meats are rich in the omega-6 LC-PUFA with 20 carbons called *arachadonic acid*.

The final form of fatty acid to explain is the *conjugated fatty acids*. Conjugated fatty acids are those that have 2 C=C's separated by a single bond. This isn't as important as realizing that they come in many isomers which contain the same number of atoms but arranged differently in structure. The most interesting one of the conjugated fatty acids is *conjugated linoleic acid* (CLA) derived from meat and dairy products. CLA comes in two common isomers, *cis-9:11* and *trans-10:12* that have unique biological properties we will further discuss.

Fats and Performance

Many studies have indicated that fish oils and CLA supplements have potential in augmenting your training in the gym. However, for every study supporting the use of these supplements there is at least one that found no effect. Athletes have been known to take these supplements to reduce body fat, increase lean muscle mass, and reduce muscle damage and inflammation. What does the science really say?

With regards to fish oil there are some theorized and realized effects of supplementation. The main theory of fish oil supplementation is that it has anti-inflammatory effect that can help limit delayed onset muscle soreness and thus get you back in the gym quicker. The omega-6 fatty acids have a pro-inflammatory effect so consuming more omega-3 fish oils tips the scales toward an anti-inflammatory environment in your body.
Ernst and colleagues demonstrated that EPA and DHA supplementation for 3 weeks reduces inflammation after an aerobic challenge. Another study on soreness after eccentric (negatives) training compared omega-3's to a placebo. They found significant reductions of

inflammatory markers in the blood of subjects immediately after and up to 48 hours after the exercise bout. Another study on eccentric bicep curls demonstrated similar findings with significant reductions in muscle soreness with 7days of 3g/d of omega-3's.

Flax seed *oil has a high proportion of omega-3 fatty acids in the form of ALA. However, your body can only convert a small percentage of the ALA consumed to the more beneficial long-chain PUFAs EPA and DHA. The omega-6 fatty acids also compete with ALA for the elongation enzyme that makes EPA and DHA. You are best off getting your EPA and DHA from fish oil and algae oil.*

Krill oil *has beneficial effects similar to fish oil in a few studies. Krill oil is derived from shrimp-like organisms found in large quantities in the ocean. Krill oil is a great source of omega-3 fatty acids. Krill has similar anti-inflammatory effects and cardio-protective benefits despite having ~60% of the EPA and DHA found in fish oil.*

Omega-3's are able to improve utilization of oxygen and flexibility of red blood cells through integration into their cell membranes. More flexible cells mean that they can squeeze their way through very small blood vessels in higher concentration carrying more oxygen to muscles. One study demonstrated that 6g/d of fish oil supplementation for 6 weeks resulted in enhanced oxygen delivery and maximal oxygen uptake during hypoxic altitude training. Beyond the clinical trials of fish oil supplementation, there are many laboratory studies that show potential benefit of fish oil on cell cultures. For instance, one study showed that DHA can enhance fat oxidation and insulin sensitivity in muscle cells. Fish oils have also been shown to increase fat oxidation, reduce bodyweight, and prevent weight gain in animal models. Even with all the laboratory and clinical evidence suggesting benefits of fish oil, a definitive answer to whether it will help your training is difficult to make. With little down side, it's worth a try in my opinion.

CLA For Fat Burning?

CLA is another fatty acid that has great results in animals, with only a few good human trials. CLA supplementation is claimed to improve body composition by helping you burn fat. Kreider and colleagues at the University of Memphis studied the effects of CLA on performance and body composition in experienced bodybuilders. Unfortunately they weren't able to demonstrate any significant beneficial effects for bodybuilders, but the study had limitations. On the contrary, studies by Thom et al. and Colakoglu et al. demonstrated that CLA supplementation improved endurance exercise performance and body composition. Furthermore animal studies demonstrate that the trans-10:12 isomer of CLA reduces fat in mice. Unfortunately natural meat and dairy sources of CLA are low in that particular isomer so use a commercial supplement for a mix of CLA isomers.

One thing bodybuilders realize is that if you want to build muscle, you must maximize your testosterone levels. Since testosterone is synthesized in your body from cholesterol, it is not a reach to realize that fats may have a role in testosterone production as well. Although research on fish oil and CLA's effect on testosterone production is still in its test-tube infancy, the studies in cell culture are promising. One study on CLA supplementation (6g/day) demonstrated very small increases in testosterone. Although fats improve testosterone production in cell cultures the mechanisms in the body seem a bit more complex.

Safflower oil has made headlines in the past year, as Doctor Oz has touted its potential to promote weight loss. Safflower oil is rich in the essential omega-6 fatty acid, linoleic acid ($\approx$78% linoleic acid). A 16 week study at Ohio State University compared high-linoleic safflower oil with CLA. The safflower oil intervention reduced belly fat and increased lean mass more effectively than CLA, although CLA did improve fat loss. However, another study suggested that substituting dietary linoleic acid in place of saturated fats increased the rates of death from all causes, coronary heart disease, and cardiovascular disease. The debate continues.

Norris LE Am J Clin Nutr. 2009 Sep;90(3):468-76
Ramsden CE BMJ. 2013 Feb 4;346:e8707

The omega-6 fatty acid arachadonic acid is thought to be beneficial for muscle building by activating protein synthesis through the signaling protein mTOR. (*See Leucine and HMB) Roberts et al. showed significant improvement in anaerobic sprint capacity with arachadonic acid supplementation. Further, data suggests that the prostaglandins from arachadonic acid are able to increase muscle cell growth via cell membrane receptors interacting with the mTOR pathway.

This is where the Goldilocks principle applies to your training. Clearly there can be too little or too much of a good thing and finding the "just right" balance is definitely a challenge for us all. Although all the fatty acids we have discussed here have potential in improving your performance supplementation will have little effect if your diet is out-of-whack. The American diet typically has ratios of omega-6 to omega-3 in excess of 10 to 1. It is theorized that humans may have evolved with a diet of a 1-to-1 ratio of omega-6 to omega-3 (Goldilocks?). The optimum ratio is thought to be at least 4 to 1 or lower for health and longevity. If you want to try fatty acid supplementation, I suggest that you begin with a clean diet with a combination of fish, lean meats, nuts, and dairy and then augment with the desired fatty acids.

Saturated Fats

The saturated fatty acids are considered the "bad fats". Clearly, lard and butter are not good for you. There are multiple studies that correlate high saturated fat intake with higher rates of cardiovascular disease. Older studies have provided evidence to recommend replacing saturated fats in the diet with PUFA's in order to reduce risk of death from heart disease. However, a study by Skeaff and colleagues in 2009 showed that saturated fatty acids may not be as bad as once thought. The research on the role of fats in your diet is complex and constantly evolving and requires consistently refreshing your knowledge base through resources like www.yourgainplan.com.
In your blood work, high total cholesterol and LDL (bad cholesterol) levels and lower HDL (good cholesterol) correlate to increased risk of heart disease, the number one killer in the

United States. There is very strong evidence that high saturated fat intake leads to higher total cholesterol, higher triglycerides, and higher levels of LDL. Other studies have correlated high intakes of saturated fats with cancer and bone disease.

Knowing that saturated fats contribute to cardiovascular disease risk, manufacturers have been replacing all fats in foods with refined simple sugars. Unfortunately, removing all fat from foods also removes some of the healthy fats that foods provide. Thus a double whammy occurs with increases in unhealthy sugars and decreases in health promoting essential fatty acids. The main thing that we should learn from studies on saturated fats is that they should only be consumed in moderation while we pay attention to including the healthy essential fatty acids, like fish oil, in a well-balanced diet. Many of the major health organizations recommend limiting saturated fat intake to less than 10% of caloric intake and even less in high risk individuals (i.e. those with obesity, diabetes, family history, smokers, etc).

Although cholesterol is produced naturally by your body, saturated fat, trans-fatty acids and dietary cholesterol can raise blood cholesterol. Monounsaturated fats and polyunsaturated fats do not appear to raise LDL cholesterol. Studies suggest that they may even help lower LDL cholesterol when eaten as part of a low-saturated and trans-fat diet. What most of this data tells us is that it really is a matter of moderate fat intake combined with a healthy ratio of PUFA & MUFA's compared to saturated and trans-fats. Eat fish, eat nuts, avocado, olive oil and avoid processed meats and treats.

Trans Fats

During food processing, oils that are unsaturated like vegetable oils may undergo a process called hydrogenation to make them more solid at room temperature like a saturated fat. This is common in margarine and shortening. These fats act similar to saturated fats raising cholesterol levels in your blood. However, the chemical processing of the fats is even more deleterious to your health than saturated fat from animal sources. Let's go over this in a little detail.

The unsaturated fatty acids can be in one of two forms "*cis*" or "*trans*." The "*cis*" form is more common in nature than the "*trans*" form. *Trans*-fatty acids are found in small amounts in various animal products such as beef, pork, and dairy fat. *Trans*-fatty acids are formed from cis-fatty acids in the hydrogenation process when making "partially hydrogenated vegetable oils". Trans-fat content is currently placed on most food labels and consumption should be limited as much as possible due to significant correlations to heart disease risk. Trans-fats lead to significant inflammation that destroys blood vessel walls leading to cardiovascular disease.

The American Heart Association's Nutrition Committee Strongly Advises:

1. Limit total fat intake to <35% percent of your total calories each day.

    I would say that in certain circumstances where you may want to be on a low carbohydrate diet, you may increase your percent calories from healthy PUFAs and MUFAs.

2. Limit saturated fat intake to <7% of total daily calories.

3. Limit trans-fat intake to < 1% of total daily calories.

   Use soft margarine as a substitute for butter, and choose soft margarines (liquid or tub varieties) over harder stick forms Look for "0g trans fat" on the Nutrition Facts label.

4. Fat should come from sources of monounsaturated and polyunsaturated fats such as nuts, seeds, fish, and vegetable oils.

   Use naturally occurring, un-hydrogenated vegetable oils such as canola, safflower, sunflower or olive oil most often.
   Look for foods made with un-hydrogenated oil rather than partially hydrogenated or hydrogenated vegetable oils or saturated fat.

5. Limit cholesterol intake to < 300mg/ day.

   If you have coronary heart disease or your LDL cholesterol level is 100mg/dL or greater, limit your cholesterol intake to less than 200 milligrams a day.

6. Choose a diet rich in vegetables, whole-grain, high-fiber foods, and fat-free and low-fat dairy most often.

   French fries, doughnuts, cookies, crackers, muffins, pies and cakes are examples of foods that are high in trans-fat. Don't eat them often.

   Limit the saturated fat in your diet. If you don't eat a lot of saturated fat, you won't be consuming a lot of trans-fat.

Limit commercially fried foods and baked goods made with shortening or partially hydrogenated vegetable oils. Not only are these foods very high in fat, but that fat is also likely to be very hydrogenated, meaning a lot of trans-fat.

Limited fried fast food. Commercial shortening and deep-frying fats will continue to be made by hydrogenation and will contain saturated fat and trans-fat.

Carbohydrates: Controlling Insulin and Inflammation

As much as diet is really all about calories in (food) and calories out (activity), controlling insulin is important to your health and maintaining a fat burning body. To reiterate, insulin is the hormone that puts us into storage mode. This is particularly important in fat and muscle. In fat, excess blood glucose is pushed into the cells by insulin and insulin turns on the machinery that makes stored fat. Insulin also shuts down the machinery that breaks the fat down. However, it is a valuable hormone when timed correctly with your workout goals as it also pushes nutrients into muscle cells to promote muscle protein synthesis. The key is limiting insulin to the small amount needed to support muscle while limiting the big prolonged spikes that generate fat. This is another "Goldilocks" zone.

We can control insulin by eating the right foods. This means a high protein, moderate fat, and low to moderate complex carbohydrate diet with very little sugar. The complex carbohydrates or "polysaccharides" require more digestion and thus take longer to absorb. Combining carbohydrates with fats, proteins, or fiber further slows their digestion and absorption. *Glycemic index (GI)* is a measure of how quickly blood glucose levels rise after eating a particular food. Foods that put glucose into your blood stream the fastest are foods with a high GI.

Eating pure sugar (glucose) has a glycemic index of 100. Pure sugar is rapidly absorbed and causes a very high rise in blood glucose and insulin. However, GI does not take into account how much carbohydrate is consumed. Glycemic Load (GL) is a measure of the total impact of a particular food on blood glucose by incorporating the quantity of carbohydrate consumed at a particular meal.

Food Labels

Having a general understanding of GI and GL is important so that you can critically analyze the foods you eat. If you look at a food label and find that the sugar content is higher than the fiber or protein content you know that food is going to raise blood glucose and insulin. If the food has more sugar on the label than complex carbohydrate it is pretty safe to say that that food will have a higher impact on your blood glucose. The more sugar there is in a food the higher the glycemic load.

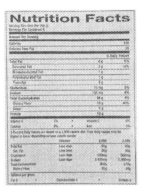 *If the food label has 25g of carbohydrate, 5g of fiber, and 10g of sugar, add together the fiber and sugar and subtract it from the total carbohydrate to get the amount of complex carbohydrate in the food.*

Further, keep an eye out for sugar in disguise: evaporated cane juice, molasses, honey, agave extract/nectar, juice concentrate, etc.

Why is it important to limit prolonged spikes in blood glucose? I briefly touched on this in the OJ Conundrum but there is more to discuss. Prolonged elevations in blood glucose lead "glycation" or caramelizing of proteins throughout the body. This results in significant damage to tissues causing systemic inflammation. This inflammation has been implicated in the formation of atherosclerotic lesions in blood vessels, heart disease, and cancer. This is the same inflammation that occurred with *trans-fats*.

Glycation of tissues like ligaments and tendons can lead to increased risk of injury. Furthermore, elevated levels of blood glucose and insulin result in other hormonal perturbations.

Chronic elevations in cortisol occur with decreased immunity and the whole host of other health problems associated with chronic stress. The conversion of thyroid hormone from T4 to the more active version T3 is reduced producing a functional hypothyroidism presenting as lower basal metabolic rate. As we discussed earlier, the worst problem is that prolonged elevations in blood glucose and insulin result in a burnout of the insulin producing cells of the pancreas and insulin resistance in tissues which results in type II diabetes.

Glycemic index is a fairly limited measure as it can vary greatly for a particular food. For instance, un-ripe bananas have a lower glycemic index than ripe bananas as the simple sugar content increases with ripening. Glycemic indexes of particular foods may differ from person to person based on speed of stomach emptying, sensitivities to foods, or changes in stomach acids or digestive enzymes. Foods that are digested more slowly gradually release glucose into the blood stream and thus have a lower glycemic index. Also, combining foods changes the absorption rate and thus affects the glycemic index of a meal. This is often a function of how much fat or fiber is in a particular meal.

Higher fat meals slow the emptying of the digesting food from the stomach to the intestines where it can be absorbed. Similarly, eating complex carbohydrates, especially in fibrous vegetables, slows the breakdown of the starch into glucose; slower digestion equals lower glycemic index. A lower glycemic response or GI of food often equates to a lower insulin response as is most often desired. In some cases the rapid rise in blood glucose afforded by a high glycemic food can be used to manipulate muscle protein synthesis via a rise in post-workout insulin.

Low GI Foods (<55):

Beans; Small Seeds; Whole Intact Grains; Vegetables, Sweet Fruits; Tagatose; Fructose

Medium GI Foods (56-69):

Not intact whole wheat or enriched wheat, pita bread, basmati rice, potato, grape juice, raisins, prunes, pumpernickel bread, cranberry juice, regular ice cream, sucrose, banana

High GI Foods (>70):

White bread, most white rice, corn flakes, extruded breakfast cereals, glucose, maltose, maltodextrins, potato, pretzels, parsnip

The glycemic index of a food is dependent on a number of factors. The type of starch or simple sugar in the food affects its glycemic index. The fat and protein content of a food affect the digestion and the rate of emptying of the food from the stomach and thus the appearance of glucose in the blood from that food. Simply adding vinegar to a meal can lower the GI of a food (apple cider vinegar goes great on salads and some meats). Additionally, the quantity of fiber in a meal or food can affect the glycemic index (See Fiber section next).

Caution must be taken when considering the glycemic index of food as the main reason for choosing a particular food. As an example, chocolate cake, ice cream, and even pure fructose have GI's less than 40! Foods like rice and potatoes may have a much higher GI. It is important to look at ingredients and ingerent nutrienta in a food. In the case of chocolate cake and ice cream, it is obvious that they are made of sugar and saturated fats. We don't need to look at the GI of those treats to know that their consumption should be moderated.

The GL is the number that correlates to how much a food will raise a person's blood glucose after a meal in relation to how much glucose is in the food. One unit of glycemic load is approximately the same as consuming one gram of glucose. The GL accounts not only for how a food raises blood glucose, but how much total carbohydrate is in the food. The GL is defined as the grams of available carbohydrate in the food multiplied by the GI/100. In other words, GL estimates the impact of carbohydrate consumption using the glycemic index while taking into account the amount of carbohydrate that is consumed. A good example of the difference in GI and GL is to look at the watermelon. A watermelon has a relatively high GI. However, since watermelon contains very little carbohydrate, the effect of eating it causes a low amount of glucose to enter the system or a "low glycemic load".(>20 considered high GL, 11-19 is considered medium and 10 or less is low glycemic load.)

The principle of GL is important to understand conceptually, but it is probably not important to focus on the actual numbers in your meals. By understanding that a food with a high GL is going to be more fat storage producing and thereby detrimental to sports performance you can tailor your diet better to achieve your goals. High GL meals are also detrimental to your health and longevity. Consistent consumption of high GL meals can lead to obesity, insulin resistance, and type 2 diabetes. Managing GL is critical for diabetics and is actually a matter of life or death.

Fruits and vegetables tend to have a lower glycemic index because of fiber content and the relatively low total amount of sugar per serving. Most fruits and vegetables (non-starchy ones) have less than 50g of carbohydrate per serving and thus testing the glycemic index of a serving compared to 50g of glucose is going to yield a low glycemic index. Further, many fruits contain fructose which is converted needs to be converted to glucose in the liver so it raises glucose levels slower. However, fructose has its own evils.

Fructose

Fructose is probably the number one source of calories in the U.S. High Fructose Corn Syrup (HFCS) is pervasive in processed foods. Normal corn syrup is mostly glucose. HFCS is corn syrup that has added fructose between 42 and 55% of its content. It is incredibly cheap for food manufacturers to utilize. Because fructose doesn't immediately stimulate insulin release like glucose, this results in a delay in the satiety of a meal. Fructose actually leaves you hungry longer and thus you eat more. It essentially tricks your body into gaining weight. Excess fructose and sugar is converted to triglycerides in the liver leading to more stored fat and increased risk of heart disease.

Fructose consumption can potentially lead to more health problems than glucose. A study from UC Davis showed significant disadvantages to fructose consumption (J Clin Invest. 2009 May;119(5):1322-34). This was an elegant study where subjects consumed 25% of their calories from glucose or fructose sweetened beverages for 10 weeks. In summary, those who had the fructose beverage showed increased rates of conversion to fat, deleterious alterations in blood lipids (increased oxidized LDL), decreased insulin sensitivity, and more abdominal (visceral) fat deposits. Without going in much more detail, fructose also seems to make cancer cells more aggressive when exchanged for glucose of culture media in the laboratory.

Fructose is clearly a bad player and should be limited as much as possible. Avoid foods with sugars and HFCS at all costs. Remember, sucrose (table sugar) found in all cane sugar including "evaporated cane juice" is half fructose! Also, beware of agave as a sweetener as it contains up to 90% fructose! Honey is also nearly 50% fructose and 50% glucose/maltose.

Supplements for Controlling Blood Glucose and Insulin

- Chromium Picolinate
- Cinnamon
- Alpha Lipoic Acid
- Vanadyl Sulfate
- CLA
- Fish Oil
- GLA
- Plant Sterol Glucosides
- White Kidney Bean Extract

My Take on Artificial Sweeteners

I have to admit, I tend to use artificial sweeteners like Splenda and Nutrasweet fairly regularly. I do this in moderation, but I have a little Splenda (sucralose) in my black coffee or with cinnamon on my oatmeal nearly every day. I believe that these are safe compounds in moderation just as the FDA would agree. However, we know that science of foods and medicine is constantly evolving and it will be important to watch for research that would change this position.

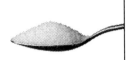

In general we eat too much sugar. We have become addicted to sweetness. To break that addiction many people need something to taper with. Just as smokers use nicotine gum and fake electronic cigarettes, some people need a little fake sweetness to wean off of sugars. In my opinion the health effects of sugars are much more deleterious than Splenda. For instance, only 15% of Splenda is actually absorbed and what is absorbed is secreted unchanged in the urine. Nutrasweet is essentially two amino acids, aspartic acid and phenylalanine. Steviol glycosides (Stevia) are naturally derived, but you may find them quite bitter. Sugar alcohols like mannitol, sorbitol, and erythritol have fewer calories, don't raise blood glucose, and don't cause tooth decay; but some people get GI side effects from their laxative effects. Saccharin is the least "natural" of the sweeteners, thus why use it at all?

As you wean off of carbohydrates and sugars in your diet you will actually find that many foods are naturally sweet. If you need sweeteners, use them moderately. Limit diet soda consumption and try water with lemon or lime wedges.

The Beef With Meat

Why is it that the media and doctors have such a "beef" with red meat? I don't have much of a beef with red meat, although there are healthier choices like fish and poultry. The problem with red meat is in the science. Many of the studies that have shown the unsavory effects of red meat on your health (heart disease, cancer, etc.) grouped together processed (bacon, sausage, lunch meats) and unprocessed meats. However, researchers at Harvard have performed an

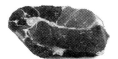

analysis of this literature and have determined that these types of meat are not created equal.

After closer evaluation of the data, the scientists demonstrated that unprocessed red meat was not significantly associated with causing more deaths; on the other hand, intake of processed meat was associated with a 30% higher rate of cardiovascular disease and cancer deaths. These findings are consistent with smaller studies showing the strong association of processed meats with cardiovascular disease. The scientists suggest that preservatives are the most notable difference. For instance, the processed meats contain up to 400% more sodium leading to greater blood pressure effects. The effects of this much sodium on blood pressure can explain the higher risk of cardiovascular disease alone.

Does red meat increase the risk colon cancer? The statistics say yes if you include processed meats and overcooked meats. It is thought that the formation of cancer causing compounds, HCA's (heterocyclic aromatic amines) and PAH's (polycyclic aromatic hydrocarbons), from meat cooked well-done at high temperatures is to blame for the increased risk. However, studies that have separated out this kind of red meat have been inconclusive and don't take into effect the lack of fiber or veggies in the diet. Fiber and veggies have been shown to be protective. Besides, frying potatoes and baking cereals creates more carcinogenic toxins (acrylamide) than overcooking meat!

Although marbled red meat is higher in saturated fat and cholesterol, lean red meat from grass-fed animals has more healthy polyunsaturated fats. Red meat also contains bioavailable forms of folate and vitamin B12. Folate and B12 are necessary to limit formation of homocysteine in your body that has been shown to be associated with cardiovascular disease and cognitive decline. In fact, homocysteine inhibits the production of the ever important nitric oxide (See Nitrates and Nitric Oxide). Meat also supplies performance and health enhancing creatine, coenzyme Q10, glutathione (antioxidant), iron, and carnosine.

In moderation, lean red meats have a place in your *G.A.I.N. Plan*. For those who are trying to grow, the extra calories and protein are useful tools. For those who need nutrient dense food, red meat is a viable option. Stick to lean red meats like venison, buffalo, ostrich, and grass fed lean cuts of beef. When caloric intake is equal, red meat is no different than chicken when it comes to "dieting". Don't be afraid to include it for the variety of nutrients.

Nitrates and Nitric Oxide

"Eat your veggies, they're good for you!" is a commonly heard mantra at dinner tables everywhere. We, the health conscious, know that veggies are good for our bodies and minds. Nevertheless, we may not know all the reasons why. It may just be that veggies provide necessary vitamins and minerals for metabolism and anti-oxidant protection. It may be that they contain colon healthy fiber to make you regular. Recent evidence suggests that it may not be the vitamins or fiber that we should be focusing on. Green leafy veggies, and the roots of the same, are rich in inorganic nitrate. Multiple epidemiological studies have demonstrated that diets rich in greens are healthy for your cardiovascular system and blood pressure. One of the hypotheses to explain this benefit is that the green leafy vegetables are rich in inorganic nitrate which acts as substrate for synthesis of blood flow boosting nitric oxide (NO). Data supports that NO is a potent booster of blood flow and cardiovascular function as you may have seen advertised in the "pump" and "vascularity" producing pre-workout "NO" supplements available to you. If you have ever tried a NO supplement, you know firsthand that they really do work.

The amino acid arginine can be converted to nitric oxide in the body by the enzyme nitric oxide synthase. In healthy conditions, added arginine isn't really necessary to maximize the function of this enzyme. However, in stressed conditions or disease states, NO boosting supplements may show benefit.

Beyond the arginine containing NO supplements, there is increasingly new data that supports the use of more direct sources of nitrogen such as nitrate as an inorganic donor for NO. Nitrate rich veggies include spinach, lettuce, celery, and beetroot. Dietary inorganic nitrate in fruits and veggies can be reduced to nitrite and nitric oxide. Some have even tried to support the use of salts of nitrates and nitrites like "salt peter" or potassium nitrate. However, a word of caution is necessary here. Although dietary nitrate is relatively safe and non-toxic, nitrite is not so safe. In fact, the toxicity of nitrite measured as its LD50 (meaning 50% of people will die at this dose) is 100-200mg *per kilogram of bodyweight*; comparable to that of cyanide! Of note, the dose of nitrate that seems to improve performance is on the order of 300-500mg, much lower than any toxic levels of nitrite. As an example, 100g of spinach may supply more than 200mg-300mg of dietary nitrate.

NO has many effects on metabolic function of blood vessels and muscle. Recent studies have suggested that nitrate supplementation might alter metabolic and vascular control of the larger, force producing type II (fast-twitch) myofibers that bodybuilders and power athletes strive to build. In mice, increases in dietary nitrate content significantly increase the rate of force development in fast-twitch muscle fibers. However, only recently have we found out that this may also occur in humans.

Scientists at the University of Exeter in the UK employed an intense exercise protocol to study the effects of beetroot juice nitrate supplementation on type II fast-twitch muscle function. the subjects were instructed to drink a total of 140 ml per day of beetroot juice for 6 days. On the testing days, they were instructed to drink the beetroot juice at least 2 hours before the exercise testing because peak levels o nitrate occur at ~2.5 hr post-ingestion. After performing the exercise protocol, researchers found that beetroot juice supplementation resulted in better tolerance of the intense exercise and better metabolic handling of oxygen than beetroot juice that was depleted of nitrate. The subjects on the nitrate rich beetroot juice took longer to fail at the high intensity sprint than those on the placebo-nitrate depleted beetroot juice.

Comparison to nitrate-depleted beetroot juice is an important aspect of this study as beetroot juice contains other potentially performance enhancing compounds. For instance, you may be familiar with betaine (beet-a-een). Betaine and polyphenols like resveratrol found in beetroot juice both have potentially beneficial effects on exercise performance. However, this study and others have found that nitrate depleted beetroot juice does not seem to enhance performance on endurance tasks or sprints.

It has long been recognized by bodybuilders that nitric oxide boosting supplements boost results from training. Many of these supplements have focused on *arginine* and *citrulline* (arginine precursor) as the precursors for nitric oxide synthesis. Recent data is now supporting that a dietary source of nitrate may also be effective in improving performance adaptations to exercise. It seems that your parents might have been right all along. Eat your veggies!

Vegetarian Diets?

Simplicity is a key to success in goal attainment. The "K.I.S.S." principle comes to mind, "Keep it Simple, Stupid!" However, living with a vegetarian diet complicates life in a meat eating society. Living on a vegetarian diet has been shown by multiple studies to be beneficial to body mass index, cholesterol, cardiovascular and cancer risks. However, this is when the vegetarian diet is well-planned and well-balanced. A poorly planned vegetarian diet can lead to muscle protein wasting, essential fatty acid deficiencies, and micronutrient deficiencies.

Humans are on the top of the food chain and our bodies are designed to consume plants *and* animals. Compared to a cow, which lives a vegetarian life, we do not have ruminating stomachs that can digest the fiber of vegetables and grains providing constant energy and nutrient delivery. Our intestines are designed to be efficient at absorbing carbohydrates, fats, and proteins. Meat, dairy, and fish provide dense and efficient sources of fat and protein. Digesting vegetables and grains for protein requires larger volumes of food and fiber as well as complex combinations of plants/grains to obtain complete proteins.

A complete protein is one that provides all the essential amino acids. Legumes are deficient in the sulfur containing and essential amino acid methionine. Grains contain methionine but are deficient in the essential amino acid lysine. Therefore, combining grains and legumes together can make a complete protein. Which is easier to make, digest, and absorb; an 8 ounce glass of milk or a big bowl of legumes and pasta? If you have time, caloric deficit, and the room in your gut eat the legumes and pasta; if not, consider the benefits of milk based whey proteins.

People who start a diet with food group restrictions usually lose some weight at the beginning. This is because one has to be very cautious about one eats and thus becomes restricted in situations where their allowed foods aren't available, such as snacking at work and eating out. As a result, the person eats less food and thus fewer calories. Vegetarians who end up skipping foods can end up with deficiencies and malnutrition. Strictly vegetarian diets (vegans) require a great deal of planning and variety in their meals. If this is appealing and sounds feasible to you feel free to be a vegetarian, it has its benefits. Multiple organizations support the heart healthy aspects of vegetarian dieting.

However, if you are a competitive athlete you may want to re-think the idea. Of course, if you have food allergies, religious restrictions, or feel a need to save farm animals live as a vegetarian and spend time planning your diet well.

Some of the problems with being a vegetarian and an athlete may be obvious. For instance, getting 1g per pound of protein (see my protein recommendations below) purely from vegetables, legumes, and grains is nearly impossible without having a bloated abdomen and/or lots of time to eat. As discussed in the chapter on proteins, inadequate protein intake and improper timing can impede progress in performance and recovery from exercise. If you are a vegetarian, consider keeping dairy foods and/or eggs included.

Another problem with vegetarian diets is creatine deficiency. Your body makes creatine from nonessential and essential amino acids in small amounts. Diet plays a critical role in supplying about ½ of the optimum creatine for athletic and mental performance. Unfortunately for vegetarians, creatine is only found in significant quantities in animals. Vegetarians have relative deficiencies of creatine compared to meat eaters which may adversely affect health by affecting brain and muscle function. An experiment described in the *British Journal of Nutrition* in 2011 looked at cognitive performance in vegetarians with and without creatine deficiency. Healthy women received daily doses of creatine or placebo for five days. The supplement, relative to the placebo, increased performance consistency and improved memory scores. This and other studies on patients with dementia suggest that creatine deficiency may reduce cognitive performance which can be reversed by creatine supplementation.

Micronutrient deficiencies can be common in vegetarians if a multivitamin or protein supplements are not consumed. Iron deficiency anemia with fatigue, weakness, shortness of breath, pale skin, and other symptoms may occur in those who don't eat meat. Vegetarians need to consciously consume iron and may even need more if they consume dairy. Dairy foods can limit the absorption of iron so iron rich foods (i.e. spinach) should be consumed with separate meals from dairy. Vitamin B-12 deficiency may also occur as it is found in meat, eggs, and milk. If you are a "lacto-ovo vegetarian" eating eggs and dairy may prevent this deficiency. Vitamin B-12 deficiency also leads to anemia symptoms with muscle weakness, fatigue, and nerve discomfort. Zinc deficiencies have been documented in vegetarians who may end up having decreases in immune function and vision problems. Another issue brought to mind by research on vegans is that they have about 6% less dense bones than those that eat meat. The lacto-ovo vegetarians showed very little difference in bone density than those who ate meat. Again, if you are thinking of becoming a vegetarian consider being a lacto-ovo vegetarian. Once your bone density decreases it can be a challenge to bring it back up as there is a gradual decline in bone density just with aging.

Vegetarians need to keep in mind the essential fatty acids. In particular, vegetarians who don't eat fish may want to consider omega-3 fatty acid supplementation via non-fish oils (i.e. flaxseed oil). There are a number of studies that espouse the multitude of health benefits imparted by fish oil consumption as we discussed. These include beneficial effects on skin, bones, muscle, blood vessels, the brain, and heart.

All that being said, vegetarians typically have lower body mass index (skinnier), serum total and low-density lipoprotein cholesterol levels, and blood pressure; reduced rates of death from ischemic heart disease; and decreased incidence of hypertension, stroke, type 2 diabetes, and certain cancers. Perhaps for the right person with time and motivation to change their life-style vegetarianism may be beneficial. *The G.A.I.N. Plan* strongly encourages vegetarians to consider all of, or some of the following: dairy, eggs, and/or fish. I also strongly recommend vegetarian athletes to consider protein, multivitamin, and creatine supplementation to help maximize performance and recovery.

Fiber and Pre-biotics

FIBER
The Essential Carbohydrate

Fiber is actually a carbohydrate that can't be digested into absorbable glucose. When you read a food label, fiber is listed under carbohydrate content and can essentially be subtracted from the total carbohydrate number to understand the glycemic load of a food. High fiber diets encourage regular bowel movements, lower blood cholesterol by preventing cholesterol absorption, decrease the risk for colon cancer, and increase longevity. Fiber rich diets have been linked to reductions in heart attacks, strokes, and diabetes.

There are 2 types of fiber; *soluble* and *insoluble*. Soluble fiber is considered a *"pre-biotic"* which means it can be fermented by gut bacteria for fuel and thus contributes to healthy gastrointestinal function. We will discuss more about the importance of your gut bacteria later in this section. Insoluble fiber is more of a "bulking" agent of food and sometimes metabolically inert without much of a pre-biotic effect. Bulking insoluble fibers attract water into the digestive system which can improve stool elimination.

Dietary fiber consists of "non-starch" polysaccharides such as cellulose, inulin, waxes, pectins, etc. In reality, the term "fiber" is a misnomer as most fiber is actually not fibrous. Plant foods contain varying degrees of soluble and insoluble fiber. For instance plums and prunes contain insoluble fiber in the skins and soluble fiber in the pulp. Both types of fiber impart health benefits. There are healthful compounds produced during the fermentation of soluble fiber and insoluble fiber improves stool bulk and transit. Sometimes the added bulk can be to a disadvantage if you are dehydrated as constipation could occur with uncomfortable bloating and gas.

It is best to consume your fiber in the form of nutrient rich vegetables, but may also be consumed as a dietary supplement. The processed root of the konjac plant has a compound similar in behavior to fiber called glucomannan. Glucomannan is sold in various forms and is often added to supplements to produce a "full" feeling which limits appetite.

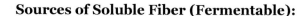

Sources of Soluble Fiber (Fermentable):

- Legumes
- Oats, rye, chia, and barley
- Fruits and fruit juices (the insides of apples and pears)
- Vegetables such as broccoli, carrots, and Jerusalem artichokes
- Root tubers and root vegetables such as sweet potatoes and onions
- Psyllium seed husk and flax seeds
- Nuts, with almonds being the highest in dietary fiber

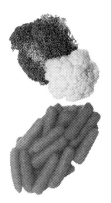

Sources of insoluble fiber:

- Whole grain foods
- Wheat and corn bran
- Legumes such as beans and peas
- Nuts and seeds
- Potato skins
- Vegetables such as green beans, cauliflower, zucchini, celery, and nopal
- Fruits including avocado, and unripe bananas
- The skins of some fruits, including kiwifruit and tomatoes

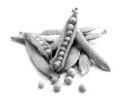

Fiber supplements are marketed for the treatment of irregular bowel movements, lowering cholesterol, reducing the risk of colon cancer, losing weight, and limiting type

2 diabetes. Soluble fiber may be beneficial for treatment of constipation and abdominal discomfort from irritable bowel syndrome. The prebiotic function of soluble fiber may also promote healthy gut bacteria that relieve symptoms of inflammatory bowel diseases like Crohn's and ulcerative colitis. Your gut bacteria can convert the soluble fiber to short-chain fatty acids that may have anti-inflammatory actions on the bowel. Some types of soluble fiber bind to bile acids in the small intestine thus making them unable to be re-absorbed later in the gut. Bile acids which are secreted to help digest and absorb fats are made from cholesterol. Thus releasing more bile acid in the stool helps rid the body of cholesterol; this explains the cardiovascular benefit of a high fiber diet.

Just the act of acknowledging the fiber content of foods may improve your diet significantly. High fiber foods tend to be wholesome and natural. Whole foods take a little more time to eat and involve more mechanical digestion by the gut. In addition to eating slower, fiber in your diet may increase the time a food is in the upper GI tract and thus attenuates the glycemic index of food. Additionally, dietary fiber interacts with digestive enzymes causing less carbohydrate to be broken down to glucose for absorption.

Healthy Colon, Healthy You:
Nutrition and Integrated Medicine

Your colon plays a couple different roles in the digestive system. The ascending or right side of the colon acts as the last chance for nutrient salvage. Gut bacteria in the right colon utilize unabsorbed starches, fats, and proteins for energy and release byproducts of these nutrients into the

GI tract. The short chain fatty acids (SCFA) that are produced by fermentation of soluble fiber in the colon play a few different roles in promoting health. Acetic acid (found in vinegar) is absorbed and enters circulation while butyric acid appears to be a preferred fuel source for colonic cells. Propionic acid enters the liver circulation and may actually have beneficial effects in reducing production of cholesterol by the liver decreasing LDL. Studies have demonstrated that SCFA's can stabilize blood glucose levels by acting on pancreatic insulin release and liver glycogen breakdown. A healthier colon lining produces a more protective barrier and better immune function. SCFAs also acidify the colon which is protective from forming colon polyps which can lead to colon cancer and improves the absorption of minerals.

A study performed by the National Institutes of Health in the 1990s demonstrated that intake of more fiber from grains resulted in a relatively lower risk of colorectal cancer. However, more recent studies have failed to show the association between fiber consumption and reduction of colorectal cancer risk. On the other hand, obesity has been linked to colorectal cancer risk and fiber rich diets have multiple benefits for obese individuals. Diets rich in dietary fiber often are less "energy dense"; that is they have less calories for a given volume of food. Thus, high fiber diets tend to lead to satiety before as many calories can be consumed in a more processed, high calorie food. The viscosity of fiber rich foods also decreases the rate of fat and glucose absorption limiting the food's impact on insulin release and triglycerides.

Consistent intake of fermentable fiber through foods like berries, vegetables, whole grains, and nuts is well known to reduce risk of the all too common diseases obesity, diabetes, high blood cholesterol, cardiovascular disease, and numerous gastrointestinal disorders. The gastrointestinal disorders include constipation, inflammatory bowel disease, ulcerative colitis, hemorrhoids, Crohn's disease, diverticulitis, and colon cancer. All of the mentioned disorders of the intestinal tract may benefit from fermentable fiber consumption.

If all that information about fiber wasn't enough, you may like to know that those who consume a diet high in fiber may benefit from it by living a longer life. That's right, dietary fiber may help you live longer. A study of almost 400,000 adults aged 50 to 71 followed for 9 years found that those who consumed the most amount of fiber were greater than 20% less likely to die in that time frame. In addition to the reduction in risk of death from heart disease, high fiber diets correlated with lower rates of infections and cancer.
The average American's daily intake of dietary fiber is well below the recommendations of all the major dietary governing bodies (i.e. ADA). The average American diet has approximately 15 grams of fiber per day compared to the often recommended 30 grams of dietary fiber per day. This lack of dietary fiber is likely due to the epidemic of processed food consumption and lack of vegetable consumption by most Americans.

One aspect of dietary fiber that is often overlooked is the caloric contribution of fiber. In the US, food labeling includes soluble fiber in the carbohydrate content of foods and considers 4 Calories per gram of fiber. However, studies suggest that because of lack of digestion and absorption in the small intestine, the amount of absorbed calories from products in the colon may be closer to 2 calories per gram of fiber consumed. This is why I don't usually include the carbohydrate content of green leafy vegetables in my calculations of macronutrient needs. Broccoli, asparagus, spinach, brussel sprouts, and lettuce are free foods in my book.

The Food and Drug Administration has given approvals for products to make health claims related to fiber content in foods. For instance, cereal producers advertises that eating their honey oats is "heart healthy" because the oat bran fiber may reduce blood cholesterol levels. As always, proceed with caution when advertisers tell you how healthy something is! The added sugar in honey oats may lead to elevated blood glucose levels, increased insulin release, elevation of triglycerides, and storage of fat.

The allowed label may state that diets low in saturated fat and cholesterol and that include soluble fiber from certain of the above foods "may" or "might" reduce the risk of heart disease.

Soluble Heart Healthy Fiber Sources Gaining FDA Approval Are:

- Psyllium seed husk - 7 grams per day

- Beta-glucan from oat bran, whole oats, oatrim, or rolled oats - 3 grams per day

- Beta-glucan from whole grain or dry-milled barley - 3 grams per day

- Functional foods and supplements include inulin, resistant dextrins, fructans, xanthan gum, cellulose, guar gum, and oligo- or polysaccharides.

Probiotics

Each of us carries more bacteria in our guts than the number of humans on the planet or the cells in your body! The metabolic activity of the more than 500 species of organisms in our gut is nearly equal to that of a vital organ. In fact some suggest the bacterial colonies in your gut should be treated like another organ system.

It can be said that the relationship between the organisms in our gut and the human body is a "*symbiotic*" relationship. This means that one organism may not be able to survive without the other. In certain situations, disruption of your gut flora can lead to severe disease and even death. The bacteria living in our intestines are useful for training the immune system, consumption of unused energy substrates (like lactose), production of vitamins, production of hormones that affect fat storage and heart disease, and protection against pathologic species of bacteria.

Probiotic bacteria and probiotic supplements have become very popular in recent years. These supplements provide large quantities of living micro-organisms that can be in even higher concentration than fermented foods and yogurt. It has been an increasingly popular way to help regulate the digestive system and presumably boost immunity to disease. Interestingly, recent evidence suggests a complex interplay between exercise, gastrointestinal physiology, and the gut microflora.

Have you ever felt nauseated or lose your appetite after a very intense workout session?

This can be related to changes in blood flow to your intestines. During exercise, our bodies our programmed to send blood to active muscles while directing blood away from restful functions like digestion in the intestines. Since the intestines experience a relative decrease in blood flow especially during a high intensity training session, there is an effect on intestinal physiology and its ability to absorb nutrients. Beyond all the beneficial effects of exercise, excessive high intensity exercise can lead to detrimental effects on the barrier properties of the intestines which block the harmful effects of pathogens. Symptoms such as bloating, cramping, and nausea may indicate an insult to intestinal barrier functions. Subsequent systemic inflammatory reactions from loss of that protective barrier function may also be detrimental to recovery from exercise and general health.

Austrian researchers examined the possibility that probiotic supplementation could protect against the detrimental effects of high intensity exercise on the GI tract. The goal of their study was to determine if multi-species probiotic supplementation improved GI barrier function and thus secondarily decreased systemic markers of inflammation and oxidation. They studied endurance trained athletes who were given a probiotic supplement in a randomized and placebo controlled double blinded fashion over the course of 14 weeks. The subjects consumed 4 grams per day of the probiotic supplement providing 2.5×10^9 colony forming units per gram. They subsequently performed a cycle ergometer exercise test to exhaustion. Blood and stool analysis was performed to determine the effects of supplementation. What the researchers found was that probiotic supplementation improved intestinal barrier function, improved markers of oxidative stress, and reduced GI inflammatory mediator TNF-a. Although most of the study data was not statistically significant, the data showed trends toward effects that may provide benefit to the immune system of athletes. One of the worst things that can happen to an athlete preparing for a competition is to end up ill and unable to train or compete.

Numerous studies suggest that probiotic supplementation may improve immune function particularly in the GI tract. Fermented foods, greek yogourt, and probiotic supplements are healthy and safe ways to boost your immune system function and potentially decrease reactive inflammation. Give the symbiotic gut flora the attention you would give any other organ in your body such as the heart or brain; feed it probiotic support. Keep your mind open as this is a rapidly evolving area of research.

Protein and Your *G.A.I.N. Plan*

The G.A.I.N. Plan should almost be called "The Protein Plan". Protein is such an important and powerful macronutrient that I believe it should be the focus of your nutrition plan. I feel that the RDA of 0.8g/kg/d for protein not only is insufficient, but produces a false impression of the importance of protein in the American diet. By suggesting that the RDA for protein is so low, the importance of protein becomes under-emphasized by most Americans. Maintaining positive nitrogen/protein balance by adequate protein intake is critical for maintaining lean muscle mass. Even non-athletes need lean muscle to maintain glucose sensitivity, basal metabolic rate, maintain bone density, and strength for day to day activities (Metabolic currency). Positive protein balance also protects the immune system and helps to heal the body from injury.

In 2004, researchers at Iowa State University, my alma mater, studied the effects of a placebo or a protein supplement given after exercise in Marine recruits. Although the supplement only had 10g of protein, it had profound effects on this population. After 54 days of basic training the protein consuming recruits had 33% fewer medical visits; including fewer viral and bacterial infections, 37% less orthopaedic injuries, and 83% less visits due to heat exhaustion. Additionally, the recruits using the protein containing supplement reported significantly less muscle soreness after training compared to control groups.

Animal studies have shown that whey protein has immune-enhancing properties. Human studies including the one above have proven that protein supplementation can help increase lean body mass, recovery after exercise, and support immune function during high-volume training periods. This is especially true when proteins containing essential amino acids are consumed before and after training sessions. If whey protein can improve recovery and immune function it can potentially help prevent over training syndrome and the subsequent attitude changes that come with it. So in essence The G.A.I.N. Plan is integrated with medicine, graded exercise, and attitude by protein.

Safety of Protein Intake

One of the biggest myths that the media and un-
informed physicians, coaches, and parents spread
is that if you consume too much protein (i.e. over
the RDA) you will have kidney problems or other
medical problems. Even when I drink protein
shakes at the hospital, other physicians ask me,
"aren't you worried about your kidneys?" I usually
say, "Did you worry about going into renal failure
with the filet you ate at dinner last night?"

For some reason, media and other outlets have
vilified sports supplements like protein shakes
and creatine into a similar category as anabolic
steroids. They make them out to be an unfair
advantage and a health risk. Fact of the matter is
that protein and creatine are beneficial nutrients
found in red meat. By media logic, one should say
that if you eat a steak you are cheating? Creatine
and protein supplements allow you to maintain a
low fat, low cholesterol diet by avoiding excessive
steak intake.

The concern that many express is that high
protein intake (by RDA standards) on a
regular basis will result in an "over working"
of the kidneys trying to filter out the break
down products of protein consumed. Over
time it is suggested that this can lead to
chronic kidney disease. The scientific evidence
that is often cited comes from animal models
where extraordinary levels of protein were
fed or human case reports in patients who
have pre-existing kidney problems. It is a big
stretch to apply these studies to the athlete
consuming extra protein. When higher
protein intakes were studied in healthy
women without kidney disease, no decline

in kidney function was found. However, in those women who had mild kidney disease, higher consumption of protein, especially non-dairy protein, lead to further decline in kidney function. Examined closer the decline in function might have been related to fat content of the meat and its effects on blood vessels and blood pressure. Even vegetarians have similar declines in renal function with age, without any protective effect of the typically lower protein intakes compared to non-vegetarians. Furthermore, clinical and epidemiological studies support benefits of a relatively high protein diet on preventing diseases that predispose one to kidney disease, such as hypertension, diabetes, and metabolic syndrome.

The International Society of Sports Nutrition also acknowledges controversy over myths that high dietary protein intake can adversely affect bone metabolism. The theory comes from studies reporting increased urine acidity from high protein intake which causes "leaching" of calcium from bone to buffer the acid. Phosphates in protein containing foods and further calcium and phosphate supplements would otherwise protect against this effect. In reality there are no studies that suggest a higher protein diet causes changes in bone density other than improvements when combined with an exercise program. The benefits of weight bearing exercise on bone density are far greater than any theoretical bone loss from added protein intake. Further evidence to support increases in protein intake by adults and the elderly for improvements in bone density is needed. Theoretically, increasing milk based protein intake may be beneficial for improving calcium and vitamin D intake as well as increasing lean body mass, both of which support healthy bone density.

The position of the International Society of Sport Nutrition is that active elderly individuals require protein intakes ranging from 1.4 to 2.0 g/kg/day, and that this level of intake is safe (ISSN Position Stand on Protein). That level is close to the 1 gram of protein per pound of bodyweight that I recommend for all athletes.

Types of Proteins and Advantages

Although my *G.A.I.N. Plan* suggests that you obtain most of your required macro and micronutrients from "whole food" sources as in a Mediterranean type diet, I am realistic about the everyday logistics of your busy life. Acknowledging the complexities of life I understand the value of nutritional supplements in simplifying performance dieting. I do recommend a relatively high amount of protein for your diet compared to the RDA at 1 gram per pound bodyweight. Getting enough protein can be difficult from whole foods during a busy schedule. Additionally, supplemental proteins like whey protein isolates have performance advantages you need to utilize.

In order to augment protein intake there are many forms of supplemental protein. These come in convenient forms such as protein bars, ready to drink shakes, powders, and pills. When it comes to pills we are usually referring to essential amino acid supplements such as branched-chain amino acids. Even though BCAA supplements can be quite useful when consumed prior to aerobic activity to spare muscle protein or even after activity to stimulate muscle protein synthesis the feasibility of using these to augment total daily protein intake is limited by sheer number of pills needed. Putting powder in a shaker cup and ready to drink shakes are very convenient and concentrated forms of protein that are very palatable and easily consumed.

Finding a good protein bar can be quite a challenge as flavors, consistency, sugar-alcohol content, and palatability can be extraordinarily variable. Sometimes the fiber content and sugar alcohol content of bars can wreak havoc on the GI tract. Sugar alcohols like sorbitol and maltitol act as osmolites and pull water into the GI tract which can cause bloating and gas. Bars are often difficult to chew and can have significant aftertaste limiting how much you can tolerate. Bars are also notorious for having inconsistent labeling of their content and often have more sugar and less protein than stated. Stick to trusted brands like GNC.

Complete vs. Incomplete Proteins

Whichever form you find more convenient the most popular forms of supplemental protein are milk proteins (whey and casein), egg protein, and soy protein. All of these types of protein are complete proteins. Complete proteins supply the body with all of the essential amino acids. These protein types are also the most digestible and deliver amino acids reliably to the muscle tissue that needs it. Incomplete proteins like lentils or wheat gluten lack certain essential amino acids and require combinations of various incomplete proteins to form a complete protein source (See Vegetarian Dieting).

Bioavailability

Protein sources have a "bioavailability" rating which describes how well it is digested to amino acids and how well those amino acids get absorbed into the blood stream. If a protein source is not very "bioavailable" then more of that protein will pass through your G.I. tract and end up wasted in your feces. The goal in consuming extra protein is to get as many essential amino acids to the muscle in an efficient and cost-effective way. Thus, I recommend sticking to the highly bioavailable sources of supplemental protein. This can have implications in pre and post-exercise training with regard to making sure that amino acids are available to stimulate muscular development and act as the building blocks of muscle (See Nutrient Timing and the Anabolic Window)

The Protein Digestibility Corrected Amino Acid Score (PDCAAS) was established by the Food and Agriculture Organization in 1991 as a scoring method which utilizes the amino acid composition of a protein relative to a reference amino acid pattern, which is then corrected for differences in protein digestibility. The U.S. Dairy Export Council's Reference Manual for U.S. Whey and Lactose Products states that whey protein isolate (derived from milk) presents the highest PDCAAS out of all of the presented protein sources due to its high content of essential and branched chain amino acids. Casein, egg, and soy protein isolate are also classified as high quality protein sources with all of them scoring a value of 1.00 on the PDCAAS scale. For a reference point, incomplete proteins like lentils and wheat gluten score a value of 0.52

and 0.25, respectively. Notably, corn protein is low in lysine and tryptophan, thus it is not a "complete protein".

For those who can tolerate milk-derived proteins, the two most popular forms of supplemental protein are whey and casein. Whey protein is separated from milk in the cheese making process. Remember Little Miss Muffett and her curds and WHEY? Casein is otherwise also derived from milk. Because of their derivation from milk those with milk allergies and lactose intolerance may have gastrointestinal difficulty with these types of protein and may need to consider egg and/or soy. The amino acid make-ups of casein and whey are more similar than egg and soy.

There is significant contrast between soy and whey. Whey has nearly 2 times the L-Threonine and ~25% more BCAAs (including leucine) than soy. Alternatively, soy has more than 2 times the L-Arginine content of whey protein. Different concentrations of amino acids may have variable effects on muscle metabolism. The literature has shown that individual amino acids can have different effects on body and muscle metabolism when supplemented independently.

Thus it can be said that all proteins are not created equal. Whether it comes from beef, milk, soy, lentils, peanuts, and so on each protein source has a different proportion of amino acids.

Whey vs. Soy

Scientists have recognized the difference between protein types and have done many comparison studies on the effects that various proteins have on body composition and recovery from resistance exercise, like weight training. Particular interest has been placed on the comparison of whey protein to soy protein.

PDCAAS of Various Proteins

- **1.00**
  Whey, Casein, Egg, Soy

- **0.92**
  Beef

- **0.91**
  Soybeans

- **0.78**
  Chickpeas

- **0.76**
  Fruits

- **0.75**
  Black Beans

- **0.73**
  Vegetables

- **0.70**
  Other Legumes

- **0.59**
  Cereals and Derivatives

- **0.52**
  Peanuts

- **0.42**
  Whole Wheat

Based on the PDCAAS whey protein, casein protein, soy protein, and egg white proteins are the complete proteins with the best digestibility. Because of this, many in the supplement industry have focused on these sources of protein when developing new products.

Other than economic reasons, comparing the two types of protein is of particular interest because whey is from an animal source and soy is, of course, a plant. Many believe the difference between these two proteins is related to the isoflavones found in soy, but research would suggest differently. In fact, in studies where isoflavone-free soy isolate was used a significant difference was still noted between whey and soy in their effects on muscle protein synthesis.

Isoflavones= estrogen (female hormone) like compounds with antioxidant properties found in legumes; also called "phyto"-estrogens or "plant derived"-estrogens.

Leucine Matters

A study reported in 2009 from McMaster University by Tang et al showed that at rest and after resistance exercise consumption of whey protein produced ~30% greater increases in muscle protein synthesis (growth) over soy supplementation. Multiple studies suggest that the BCAA L-leucine has stimulatory effects on muscle protein synthesis and whey protein has nearly 30% more leucine than soy.

A 2014 study by Mamerow et. al. (*JNutr*) showed that most people eat their protein skewed toward the end of the day with 10g at breakfast, 15g at lunch, and up to 65g at dinner. When they evened out the protein consumption to 30g with each meal they found higher total daily muscle protein synthesis amounts. Thus, some threshold to maximize muscle protein synthesis was not being reached at each meal. I propose that this threshold was the amount of leucine needed to turn on muscle protein synthesis. As we will discuss in the 5-MAD section, 3 meals per day can be improved upon as well.

Leucine is a particularly important branched-chain essential amino acid. Leucine has many beneficial affects to you as an athlete and a dieter. Leucine does a few things:

1. Leucine turns on muscle protein production. In other words, leucine turns on the muscle growth machinery. Leucine turns on muscle production by acting through similar path ways as insulin, the mTOR pathway. It has been demonstrated that consuming 0.04-0.05mg of leucine per kilogram bodyweight per meal can maximize muscle protein synthesis. Thus, I recommend that you attempt to maximize the leucine content of your meals. *The G.A.I.N. Plan* diet app for the iPhone will help you to recognize the leucine content of your foods and how this relates to your needs.

2. Leucine is the anti-glucose. First of all, leucine is an amino acid that can't be converted to glucose via gluconeogenesis. It is one of only 2 amino acids that don't convert to glucose (the other is lysine). Second, leucine has the ability to boost insulin production and insulin sensitivity in order to help clear the toxic glucose from the blood.

3. Leucine metabolites help to prevent breakdown of protein. Leucine can be converted to beta-hydroxy-beta-methylbutyrate (HMB) and alpha-keto-isocaproic acid (KIC). Both of these compounds, particularly HMB, limit the

breakdown of proteins. This is why I recommend consumption of 3g of HMB and BCAA's prior to your fasted cardio training, to spare muscle.

One myth that comes up often is that your body can only absorb 20-30g of protein per meal anyway. If this was the case, it would be very hard to reach the 0.04mg/kg of leucine per meal. This myth evolved from studies saying that 20g of protein or essential amino acids maximizes muscle protein synthesis. However, those studies did not evaluate the effect of consuming more protein on limiting muscle protein breakdown. Muscle protein is in constant flux with synthesis and breakdown. Activity tries to break it down and the body has to build it up in rest and recovery. If you consume more protein it will actually help limit muscle breakdown. So don't hold back because of incomplete science.

Despite individual metabolism and performance variables, I would like to make some steadfast recommendations about your protein intake:

1. **Consume more than adequate amounts of protein.**
   Protein consumption is safe if you are healthy and have normal kidney function. The worst case scenario is to be in negative nitrogen balance and be losing hard earned muscle because you are not consuming as much protein as you need. Try to maintain at or near 1g of protein per pound of your body weight.

2. **Consume a variety of proteins.**
   Variety is important in every aspect of your training including your diet. Consuming a variety of proteins such as fish, eggs, meat, and dairy will help provide a variety

of micronutrients and fats that are essential to health, longevity, and performance.

3. **Timing of your protein is important.**
   Try to maintain a steady source of blood amino acids by eating meals ~every 3 hours. (See the 5MAD diet) Spike the system with 3-6g of leucine by consuming high quality protein such as a whey isolate (+/-casein) before and after your workouts. This will maximize muscle protein anabolism, prevent catabolism, and take advantage of the anabolic window around your training session.

4. **Even endurance athletes need protein!**
   You are what you eat and if you don't eat enough protein you won't have enough muscle. Maintaining muscle mass is critical to the endurance athlete. This is done by consuming adequate amounts of muscle sparing protein and energy boosting carbohydrates and fats.

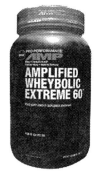

5. **Consider a combo protein supplement with both Casein and Whey Isolate.**
   This will likely cover your bases with regards to rapid and slowly absorbed protein as well as promotion of muscle protein synthesis. If you have intolerances, soy or egg proteins are possible alternatives. Regardless of which protein supplement you use, using one is better than not having the protein at all. Will the difference in your physique or performance be affected by which of the 4 protein supplements you choose? Only you can answer that by experimenting with them yourself.

a. Try micro-filtered whey isolate first as it is relatively lactose free, easily mixes, and is quite palatable as a shake, in cereal, in oatmeal, or in cooked foods. It is a consistent product and intermediate in expense.

b. If available a combo protein of micro-filtered whey isolate and hydrolysate is very palatable, mixes well, and has the advantage of rapid amino acid absorption with both micro-fractions and bi- and tri-peptides that can be biologically active.

c. If cost is prohibitive and you can tolerate lactose, fat, and cholesterol whey protein concentrates still have the beneficial effects of its BCAAs, micro-fractions, and favorable digestibility of whey.

d. If you choose soy protein, consider adding leucine and the other BCAAs to boost the effects on muscle protein synthesis.

(See the yourgainplan.com blog for more information on the various types of whey protein)

Nutrient Timing: The Anabolic Window

In order to gain muscle and lose fat you must have adequate nutrients available to do so. Not only do you need nutrients as building blocks for the muscle itself, but also as an "on" switch for the muscle producing machinery in your body. Your muscles act like are a power plant. If there are adequate amounts of coal to burn (glycogen), sufficient demand for power (exercise), and good management of the facilities (amino acids and hormones) the plant will be productive (build muscle).

We have already discussed the importance of exercise intensity in stimulating muscle growth. However, if the demand is too high (as in overtraining) the power plant doesn't keep up and the plant burns out or breaks down. The management gets frustrated and the system goes into chaos. In the body that management includes anabolic and catabolic hormones. Anabolic hormones are those that stimulate muscle growth, while catabolic hormones are counter-productive by breaking down muscle. When the system is over-stressed catabolic hormones like cortisol become elevated and muscle growth and healing are hindered.

The hormones that promote muscle growth include, but aren't limited to, IGF-1, growth hormone (GH), testosterone, and insulin. These anabolic hormones respond to the availability of nutrients and stimulus for growth (intense exercise). When present, these hormones turn on the muscle building machinery. That machinery is activated for up to 48 to 72 hours after a workout. If too much stimulus is added to the machinery within that time the machines get overloaded and can't keep up with demand. As a result, muscle fails to grow and setbacks can occur with injuries (overtraining syndrome).

After a workout, there is a well-documented "anabolic window" in the first 3 hours. This is a time when your muscle cells are extra sensitive to nutrients and hormones. Muscle preferentially converts nutrients to new muscle proteins during this time. Insulin is a hormone that responds to blood glucose levels and protein (albeit greater to glucose). This is the hormone that lets nutrients into the muscle cell, the gatekeeper if you will.

CARBS NOT REQUIRED

It is often said that this is the most anabolic hormone in the human body. Without insulin (type I diabetes) muscle can't grow because very little nutrients would be available for building the muscle proteins. Insulin is the manager that essentially says there are enough coal cars to run the power plant. This manager signals the furnace doors to open and turns on the plant. That is, insulin causes glucose and amino acids to be brought into the muscle cell while turning on muscle protein synthesis machinery. The more glucose available the higher the insulin levels in your blood. Amino acids, although to a lesser degree, stimulate a rise in insulin thus turning on the machinery as well. In particular, the branched-chain amino acid leucine acts as a messenger for the manager (insulin) to also activate muscle protein synthesis machinery. However, leucine doesn't need insulin to have the same effect so this can be done *without* carbs. During exercise and shortly after, your muscle cells are leaky and let glucose in without the need for insulin. This can be taken advantage of as well.

What to consume after your workout has been a subject of much debate. The answer to this question is quite dependent on your goals, daily caloric needs, the macronutrient makeup of your diet, and the type of exercise or sport you perform. Endurance sports expend a great deal of calories. In order to maintain energy balance and avoid losing valuable muscle your caloric intake must be equal to or greater than your energy expenditure. If you are doing endurance exercise to lose weight, then expect that you may lose some muscle with this if your energy output is greater than intake. The muscle loss can be minimized with optimization of nutrients during the anabolic window. If your endurance training is meant to build endurance and speed you must fuel the machinery to build and restore.

When trying to lose weight one would want to avoid consuming too many carbohydrates. Carbohydrates, in particular simple sugars, stimulate insulin release and thus the absorption and storage of excess nutrients. Insulin also shuts down the machinery that burns fat so that the machinery that stores fat can get to work. Thus consuming sugars or significant amounts carbohydrate after your training will limit the activation effect of the training on fat burning machinery. If you avoid carbohydrates immediately after a fat burning workout, you will continue to burn fat longer. However, endurance training for performance depletes stores of glucose (glycogen) needed for energy to feed working muscles. If your goal is to maximize performance and even build some muscle, adding carbohydrates to stimulate insulin release will help replenish the muscle glycogen and turn on the protein synthesis machinery. Leucine rich protein in post-workout (i.e. Whey isolates) would be a nice intermediate with slight rise in insulin while not so much to inhibit fat burning.

If excess carbohydrate is consumed it will be stored as fat. Amino acids in the blood that arise from consuming proteins produce a much smaller insulin response and is actually is balanced out by a similar rise in the counter-balancing catabolic hormone glucagon. Glucagon acts to mobilize glucose stores into the blood to raise blood glucose levels. Thus a protein meal with less carbs helps prevent storage of glucose as fat. In an athlete looking to build muscle and burn fat, a lower carbohydrate diet and high protein intake is important to maximize the hormonal milieu and protein synthesis.

Now, depending on how quickly you are trying to lose weight the anabolic window can be manipulated in different ways. If you are trying to lose fat relatively quickly with less interest in maintaining your muscle mass, elimination of insulin stimulating carbohydrates is in your interest. However, if you are on a much more gradual fat loss and muscle sparring program (which I prefer you do), maximizing the anabolic window while decreasing insulin stimulation through the rest of the day is important. The anabolic window is the best time to add carbohydrate to your diet as the likelihood that your muscle converts your nutrients to muscle preferentially over fat is greater. Exercised muscle likes to fuel muscle protein synthesis preferential to fat storage. Thus, if you are consuming *any* carbohydrates it is best done after your resistance training. Keeping your carbohydrate levels low throughout the rest of the day allows for lower insulin levels and thus lower activity of fat storing machinery.

Healthy Diet:
The 5 Meal A Day Plan (5-MAD)

Your body needs a regular and consistent supply of nutrients to build and recovery from intense exercise. The typical 3 meals per day of breakfast, lunch, and dinner just doesn't fit our physiology. By the time lunch comes around, assuming you had a good breakfast, you are probably very hungry. Somewhere along the way you may have already had a snack to quench those hunger pangs. Often times that snack is inappropriately some over-processed, sugar laden, malnutritious food that you pulled out of a bag or machine, just to "hold you over". Recall the OJ Conundrum?

In reality, that snack just made things worse for lunch. The highly processed and rapidly absorbed carbohydrates in your snack result in an insulin surge that causes a rapid decline in blood glucose and worsening of your appetite. You go into lunch with a desire to eat as much if not more food and you get that wonderful post-lunch slump in energy. This is a vicious cycle that can be broken by re-thinking your eating schedule.

I suggest that you adopt a 5 meal a day plan (5MAD) to stabilize blood glucose levels and supply your muscle with quality nutrients and leucine throughout the day. Studies on maximizing muscle protein synthesis and even feeding schedules in critically ill patients suggest an every 3 hour meal plan. We already discussed the importance of low-glycemic carbohydrates, high quality proteins, and essential fatty acids. Each meal should keep these in mind while supplying fiber and antioxidants preferentially from nuts or veggies. More importantly, each meal should contain essential nutrients that you can't live without. Again, there are essential amino acids in protein, essential fatty acids in fats, and essential vitamins and minerals in nutrient dense foods. There are no essential carbohydrates, so starches and sugars are not absolutely necessary in every meal.

In sports training or in those just trying to lose body fat meal frequency and nutrient timing are very important in maintaining performance goals. The typical 3 meal per day, breakfast, lunch, and dinner just doesn't cut it when trying to maximize performance. Depending on how long your day is a 3 meal per day plan leads to excessive periods of time without fuel to recover and build muscle during training.

During infancy, babies tend to eat more meals throughout the day. Have you ever noticed how quickly a baby doubles their bodyweight and size? They are rapidly growing consuming milk protein on a more frequent schedule than 3 meals per day. If you want to grow and put on muscle, eat more like a baby! Human breast milk is very high in whey protein (60:40 Whey to casein, Cow's milk is 20:80). Nature has decided that whey is the way to grow!

Increasing meal frequency does not have a beneficial effect on total body fat in itself. Some think that increasing meal frequency without changes in calorie intake can increase metabolic rate and thus fat burning, but this isn't supported by the scientific literature. However, if your protein intake is adequate, increased meal frequency has the ability to help you spare muscle mass when in an energy deficient fat burning program; i.e. when calories in are lower than calories expended. At least, 30 grams of protein per meal (15g of essential amino acids or 3 to 6g of leucine) will optimize muscle protein synthesis in most people. More meals with protein less than this will result in deficits in maximizing muscle protein synthesis and repair. Larger amounts of protein are needed with each meal to maximize its effect. Your muscle's effectiveness in burning fat may also be improved by having smaller meals as less insulin is released

at a given meal. Insulin shuts down fat burning
and switches on fat storage.

A snack between meals has actually been shown to
burn more body fat and improve strength despite
small increases in total calories consumed.

Beyond the muscle sparing effects of eating more
than 3 meals per day, the increase in frequency
improves appetite control and limits hunger.
When we say eating more than 3 meals per day we
do not mean that you eat your usual 3 meals and
add meals on top of that, such that you are eating
more calories. If you goal is to gain weight, this
might be the case. But in the situation where you
are trying to maximize performance or trying to
burn fat, the goal is to maximize the effects
of meal frequency in limiting hunger and
muscle breakdown.

Also, an increase in meal frequency has beneficial
effects on blood markers of health such as
cholesterol and even decreases blood pressure.
Eating greater than 4 meals per day with the
same total calories as someone eating 3 meals
per day can lead to lower total and bad LDL
cholesterol levels. The effect is almost as strong
as some pharmaceutical interventions for high
cholesterol! Consuming less food in one setting
also decreases the amount of insulin released
such that the potential for storing nutrients and
decreasing sensitivity to insulin doesn't occur.
Without excessive levels of blood glucose less
"caramelizing" of tissues occurs and thus less total
body inflammation.

Peri-exercise Nutrients

During moderate intensity exercise glycogen stores (stored glucose in muscle) are limited to a few hours if you are well fed. As those levels of stored glycogen decrease, performance decreases proportionately. When glycogen stores are depleted muscle tissue breakdown and immune system dysfunction can occur. This has been the prevailing motivation behind carbohydrate loading before exercise, especially endurance exercise. Research evaluating the performance effects of ingesting carbohydrate prior to exercise has shown that carbohydrate ingestion routinely improves use of carbohydrate for energy. Studies overwhelmingly suggest that this either maintains a consistent level of performance or may slightly improve it.

Ingestion of protein or essential amino acids prior to exercise alone or in combination with carbohydrate has been scientifically evaluated. Combining whey protein with carbohydrate improves muscle protein synthesis when ingested immediately before exercise. The protein synthesis rates during recovery from resistance exercise can remain elevated for 3 hours after exercise and are improved by protein and carbohydrate consumption. A study by scientists from Australia demonstrated a profound benefit to supplementing protein, creatine, and carbohydrate immediately before and after a workout versus consuming the same supplement in the morning and evening (not immediately around the workout time). Supplementation with protein, carbohydrate, and creatine produces greater increases in lean body mass, 1 repetition maximum strength, muscle size and higher muscle creatine and glycogen levels. Scientists have demonstrated that consumption of supplements containing carbohydrate, fat, and protein (chocolate milk for instance) can improve vertical jump power and number of repetitions of high intensity resistance training when ingested within 30min prior to the exercise.

There is another aspect of pre-workout nutrition that deserves recognition by the gain plan. Caffeine supplementation prior to exercise or competition. Caffeine is effective in improving performance in trained athletes at moderate doses around 2 mg per pound bodyweight (about as much as a bold grande Starbucks coffee). Caffeine supplementation can improve performance in endurance exercise and high intensity intermittent exercise like soccer or rugby. Caffeine can even improve concentration during exercise and recovery from training. One fear about caffeine is that it may have a "diuretic" effect that can lead to dehydration and a subsequent detriment to performance. However, this effect is not supported by the scientific literature and caffeine use appears to be safe.

Intermittent Fasting: A New Perspective On Ancient Physiology

Modern humans are still genetically adapted to a pre-agricultural hunter-gatherer life-style. Our overall genetic makeup has changed very little during the past 10,000 years. Hunter-gatherer societies likely had to undertake moderate physical activity for certainly more than the currently recommended 30 minutes each day to provide basic necessities, such as food, water, shelter, materials for warmth, and so forth, to survive.

One might deduct that any gene that didn't support an active lifestyle would have resulted in natural selection of that gene to die off. On the other hand, a gene that would support physical activity even in times of famine would have been more likely to survive, and its gene pool would be inherited by future generations. Thus it is likely that many metabolic functions of modern humans evolved as an adaptation to a physically active lifestyle, coupled with a diet high in protein and low in carbohydrate, interspersed with frequent periods of famine.

The concept of cycles of feast and famine engendered Neel's "thrifty gene" hypothesis. According to this hypothesis, those individuals with "thrifty" metabolic adaptations would convert more of their calories into fat during periods of feasting. As a consequence, those with the thrifty genes would be less likely to die off during food shortages because they had better fat stores. This theory certainly has its critics but it helps us to understand some of our modern physiology.

A reduction in energy intake below your body's requirements results in a series of physiological, biochemical, and behavioral responses, which are an adaptation to the low-energy intake. Once the body burns off all of its stored glucose (glycogen) it starts to burn fat for energy. In times of prolonged energy restriction muscle is broken down into amino acids that can be used for energy production. Furthermore, when energy intake is low, your behavior becomes one of less energy output; you become less active and your metabolism slows down. Because inactivity also produces muscle atrophy, we can speculate an evolutionary origin for the selection of genes that turn muscle growth on or off based on availability of nutrients.

When we chronically energy restrict our diets as in a weight loss program we turn on some of these adaptive responses. Our metabolism has a tendency to slow down, we stop building muscle or even lose muscle, and we have a greater tendency to store extra food as fat. This leads to the problems of the Yo-Yo dieter. When we restrict food for a significant period of time, we lose our muscle which acts as metabolic currency. The more muscle we have the more fat burning potential we have. When the dieter who has lost muscle goes back to eating more than they need, they end up storing more fat because the fat becomes a sponge and the muscle is gone.

Many are now realizing that chronically restricting energy intake is probably not the best way to burn fat. Although there are animal studies that suggest that lower energy intake leads to longer life, this has yet to be convincingly proven outside the controlled laboratory environment or in primates. Chronic energy restriction leads to hormonal changes, reduced muscle mass, lower bone density, increased risk of infection, susceptibility to biological stress, and increases in food seeking behavior. This is where the concept of intermittent fasting comes into play.

I have always utilized fasting physiology in my contest preparation to burn fat while sparing my muscle mass. I did this through a high protein, low carbohydrate diet with healthy fats and utilization of fasting morning cardiovascular exercise. By avoiding carbohydrates in my last

2 meals and an overnight fast of 8 hours sleep, my glycogen stores were minimized by morning. By doing fat burning cardio in this state, my body would have to search for other sources of energy than stored glucose. The next preference is to burn fat. With use of muscle sparing supplements like branched-chain amino acids and HMB I burned fat while maintaining my metabolic currency.

Intermittent fasting (IF) has potential to be a better way to burn fat and stay healthy than chronic caloric restriction. IF comes in many forms and techniques. Some IF techniques involve an entire day of fasting only allowing tea, coffee, or water. I'm not one to encourage such techniques. Another technique is to have a significantly energy restricted day twice per week where one only eats a small amount of food with less than 50g of carbohydrate. Others recommend fasting for the first half of the day skipping breakfast and working out while fasted. Some techniques just recommend a 6 to 8 hour window of eating to get your daily needs.

IF puts the body on notice that glucose won't always be available to burn for fuel. In diets where you eat throughout the day with the typical RDA of carbs over protein and fats the body is constantly using glucose for fuel. By fasting you encourage fat burning machinery to stay active and ready to mobilize fat from its stores.

IF has been proven by science to be as effective if not more effective in helping subjects lose weight and restore insulin sensitivity than chronically energy restricted diets. Insulin's job is to clear glucose from the blood by driving it into tissues like muscle and fat. Regular intake of sugar causes elevated release of insulin that the body can become resistant to. Type II diabetes is a result of a loss of sensitivity to insulin that causes blood glucose levels to rise. This leads to higher risk of heart disease and cancer. Type II diabetes is thought to be a result of "thrifty genes" that were used by the body to keep blood glucose levels higher in times of famine to fuel the brain with glucose. IF seems to restore normal physiology in overweight individuals by burning fat and restoring insulin sensitivity. IF also improves blood triglyceride and cholesterol levels further reducing the risk of heart disease.

Short episodes of fasting help train your body to deal with stress. Exercise and fasting affect your physiology in similar ways. By forcing your body to use other sources of energy, i.e. fat, IF trains your body to burn fat more efficiently. The metabolic engines of your muscle respond to stress much like they respond to weight training. If you give the muscle stress by lifting heavy weight it tends to grow. However, if you over stress the muscle with too much weight or too much energy restriction, you induce an overload that can do more harm than good. Thus, proponents of IF don't suggest that you fast forever, but that you do it in small bursts.

IF also seems to normalize other hormones. Growth hormone is a restorative hormone that is released in response to exercise and sleep. It plays a role in maintaining muscle mass while also maintaining blood glucose levels and mobilizing fat to be burned. Fasting has been shown to temporarily raise growth hormone levels by as much as 1300% in women and 2000% in men.

Perhaps this is a good way to burn fat while preserving muscle mass? IF also normalizes hormones that lead to hunger thus it becomes less difficult to deal with the lack of food. The "hunger hormone" ghrelin is reduced by IF.

One more benefit that is worth mentioning is the effect of fasting on the brain. In animals that are stressed by a lack of food, their brains become more active to help them focus on finding food. Furthermore, the brain likes ketones that arise from the breakdown of fat for fuel. Studies show that alternate day fasting where the subject consumes only 600 calories in one meal on the fasting day increases brain-derived neurotrophic factor (BDNF) by up to 400%. BDNF is involved in the growth of new brain cells and learning. Studies also show that exercise is associated with similar increases in BDNF. Further, this elevation in BDNF is thought to be protective in cognitive diseases like Alzheimer's Dementia. In animal models, IF can delay the onset of memory disorders like Alzheimer's.

So if this convinces you to try IF, you are in for a challenge. Most studies of IF have a pretty high attrition rate. This means that they were very difficult diets to follow and many just couldn't hack it for the full 12 week study. I would recommend starting with a 5:2 diet. This is 5 days of regular eating with 2 days interspersed where you only eat an afternoon meal of restricted calories. For instance, you eat basically what you want for 2 normal days at 2000 calories, and then eat only 600 calories for one afternoon meal and alternate accordingly. I would consult with your physician before trying any new diet routine, especially one this radical.

My thoughts are that you don't have to do a full fast of such extremes to get the effects of fasting. A low carbohydrate and high protein diet with the timing of your meals around your exercise can have similar effects. Try doing fasted morning cardio and train weights in the afternoon after you have had a couple meals and a pre-workout shake. Have your BCAAs and HMB to help spare muscle and keep your protein intake up to at least 1g per pound bodyweight. Eat a well-balanced diet with veggies, fish, meats, eggs, nuts, and dairy; or just go Paleo if you want to live like your cave-dwelling ancestors!

G.A.I.N. Plan Diet Implementation

The G.A.I.N. Plan diet is based on scientific evidence to match your goals. Whether you want to lose weight, gain muscle, or just live healthy the *G.A.I.N. Plan* diet will guide you along the way. To simplify your life, yourgainplan.com can guide you through making the diet program to achieve your goals. You may find yourself fitting into one of 3 categories:

1. **Health Maintenance**

   You feel that you are at your ideal bodyweight and you want to maintain that weight while living healthy for longevity. The focus is on balanced nutrition to support your desired level of activity. This category is for those who like to take a holistic approach to their longevity.

2. **Muscle Gainers**

   This category is for those of you that want to build muscle for bodybuilding or performance. This can also be for those who want to improve their endurance performance. Muscle is metabolic currency and this category needs more energy and fuel to build. Gain as much muscle as you need and fuel your competitive spirit.

3. **Fat Burners**

These folks are desiring to lose the extra fat weight while maintaining as much muscle as possible. You may be preparing for a physique competition. You might need to make weight for a sport. You may need to lose weight because your doctor told you. Losing weight means that you'll be burning fat and possibly losing some muscle. There are no miracles here. A proper diet and the right amount of exercise and you will burn the fat.

The G.A.I.N. Plan diet is based on a number of scientific principles in order to maximize your lean muscle mass while losing fat or beefing up. The goal of any category above is to stay anabolic and maintain your "metabolic currency" called muscle. Losing weight is largely a catabolic process, but anabolic stimuli can still help you to maintain muscle while losing the fat. The diet helps you to maintain your muscle by doing a few things:

1. **It Avoids the Starvation Response.**

The G.A.I.N. Plan diet employs calculations and real-time biometric measurements of your daily caloric expenditure to make sure that you are getting enough calories for your goals. If you are trying to burn fat I recommend that you produce most of your caloric deficit through added exercise while limiting your caloric deficit from food.

I recommend that you should never restrict more than 250 Calories from your diet and your total energy deficit should not exceed 500 Calories (250 from food and 250 from exercise. Exceptions may apply in cases of health risks. With an emphasis on healthy fats, protein, fibrous veggies, and nutrient timing you will feel fuller and less "starved" than on other more restricted diet programs.

2. Maximizes Protein Intake.

The ACSM and ADA recommend 0.8 grams of protein per pound for strength and endurance training athletes. On the 5MAD diet this comes out to 24 grams of protein per meal for a 150 lb man. Unfortunately, this is just not enough protein to supply necessary amino acids for maximizing muscle maintenance. Particularly, as will learn below, this is not enough protein for maximizing leucine delivery. My personal experience and science supports the use of substantially more protein to maximize muscle growth and prevent breakdown in dieting. Sometimes you need to reduce your carbohydrate and fat intake to maximize fat burning. In this case, you will go into starvation mode without the addition of protein for calories. Increasing the proportion of calories from protein increases metabolism and improves mobilization of fat stores. If you have any question of the safety of such a diet, consult your physician (See Protein Safety). *The G.A.I.N. Plan* diet includes no less than 1 gram per pound bodyweight per day.

3. Provides Adequate Leucine at Each Meal.

Leucine is an amazing amino acid. It is a branched-chain amino acid that acts as a signal for your muscle to build muscle when adequate nutrients are present. Studies show that the leucine content of a protein affects its ability to boost muscle protein synthesis, especially after exercise. Studies also support that leucine can maximize muscle protein synthesis with at least 0.04 grams per kilogram of bodyweight per meal (adjusted to reach 1.8g minimum for 100lb person). The proteins and supplements recommended by *The G.A.I.N. Pla*n diet are intended to meet that need with each meal.

4. **Maximizes Your Antioxidant and Micronutrient Intake.**

Through the use of fibrous and green leafy veggies, *The G.A.I.N. Plan* diet maximizes your intake of vitamins and minerals that are needed to recover from workouts. The vitamins, minerals, and antioxidants from whole foods are very well absorbed. Veggies are also rich in nitrates that help to deliver valuable nitric oxide. Nitrates improve performance, increase delivery of oxygen and nutrients to muscle, and help control blood pressure.

5. **Gives You Goal Oriented Supplement Advice.**

Nutritional supplements are essential to the success of your *G.A.I.N. Plan*. When you aren't able to maximize your protein and leucine content of a meal through whole foods (especially due to caloric restrictions, food volume, or meal time limitations) supplements become a savior. A multivitamin ensures you that you have fulfilled your micronutrient needs. Some supplements are essential to compete on the athletic stage. Supplements like creatine, beta-alanine, arginine/citrulline, and betaine boost strength and muscle endurance leveling the playing field. Some supplements help you to increase your metabolic rate and burn more fat throughout the day. There are many out there with and without science to back them up. I will direct you the right way.

Figure Out Your G.A.I.N. Plan Diet

By following the algorithm below, you can create the best diet for attaining your goals. Adjust the diet weekly depending on your progress, attitude, energy level, and health. The app at yourgainplan.com will automate and simplify this process. Sugars, desserts, and alcohol are never included in *The G.A.I.N. Plan* diet. If you add these you'll need to make up for it through added exercise or reductions in carbohydrate or fat calories.

1. Once your total daily energy expenditure is calculated based on your *G.A.I.N.* Monitor weekly average or use of BMR calculators like those found at yourgainplan.com (Harris-Benedict Equation) you have a starting point for the diet. These equations only require your height, weight, age, and sex. This calculation is done using your *goal weight*. More accurate assessments can be done if you know your body fat percentage. When setting up a goal we start with [BMR x 1.2]. 1.2 is the activity factor for a sedentary individual. This gives us a baseline on to which we add or subtract calories in the form of foods or exercise.

Calculate Your BMR x 1.2 via the Harris Benedict Equation on page 258

_____

_____

_____

_____

_____

_____

_____

Make life easy, use the G.A.I.N. Plan App!

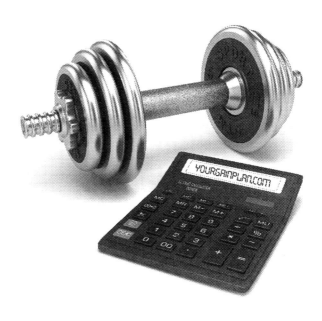

2. With the total daily energy expenditure calculated you can now determine your macronutrient needs.

a. Your protein intake will be a minimum of 1 gram per pound and enough to generate 0.04g/kg of leucine

b. Subtract the number of calories obtained from 1g/lb of protein from the total daily expenditure (grams of protein x 4 Cal/gram). BMR – (4 x Bodyweight) = calories left over after protein met

c. After the protein calories have been subtracted we divide the remaining calories into fat and carbohydrate calories based on your goal category.

   i) Health Maintenance. Divide the remaining calories 50/50 between carbs/fats

   ii) Muscle Gainers. Divide the remaining calories 60/40 carbs/fats

   iii) Fat Burners. Divide the remaining calories 40/60 carbs/fats

d. Next, you need to make adjustments based on your goal.

   i) Health Maintenance. Depending on your level of physical activity you add calories evenly distributed between carb/protein/fats to match your daily energy expenditure in exercise. Your meals can be planned with the sedentary activity level and nutritious foods can be added ad lib to match your level of calorie expenditure in exercise. This is preferred in the form of nuts, veggies, lean meats, or protein bars/shakes/supplements.

ii) Muscle Gainers. Your added calories from exercise will be added to your sedentary baseline by equal distribution into carbs and protein 50/50. It is recommended that 250 Calories be added on top of your baseline sedentary calories and exercise calories. This will ensure you that you have plenty of calories to remain anabolic. Note: if you add more than 250 extra calories chances are you will put on fat weight. If this is OK for your goal, feel free to do this with extra protein, healthy fats, or complex carbohydrates.

iii) Fat Burners. I recommend removing no more than 250 Calories from the diet. These calories are removed equally from carbohydrates and fat. Your remaining caloric deficit should come in the form of exercise. If your deficit is more than 500 Calories per day you run the risk of significant muscle loss and a slowing of your basal metabolic rate with the starvation response. Slow and steady weight loss is always better than rapid weight loss (with only few exceptions such as morbid obesity).

3. Now that you have your calories divided into each macronutrient, divide each by their Calorie content to get the number of grams to be consumed (divide by 4 for protein and carbs, 9 for fats).

4. With the total grams of each macronutrient divide each equally over 5 meals (5MAD). After you select your protein sources it is at this point when you can determine if your

leucine content is high enough per meal. If it isn't you need to make one of these adjustments to meet your needs:

a. Add supplemental leucine. Often just adding 1 gram of leucine to your meal will suffice. This will not count toward daily calories

b. Add supplemental protein to meals. This can be done in the form of added lean protein (chicken, fish, lean meats, whey/casein/soy/egg protein). In the *Fat burners*, remove the added calories of added protein from fat and carbohydrates equally. In the *Muscle Builders* accept the extra protein calories without any other changes.

5. Now that you have the macronutrient requirements for each meal, select your favorite foods from the *G.A.I.N. Plan* preferred food list available at yourgainplan.com.

6. Additional snacking will need to be considered by the diet or added exercise. As you have learned in the book, sugar is the enemy to success. Limit fruits to essential timing; i.e. add as post-workout carbs or during intense training/competition sessions. Snacking should come in the form of nuts and fresh fibrous veggies; almonds, cashews, walnuts, pistachios, pecans, broccoli, cauliflower, celery, etc. It is preferred that snacking is avoided as much as possible as you should be able to stick to the 5MAD diet which means meals are every 3 hours.

7. Condiments should be used in a complimentary way. If you are in the health

maintenance category, utilize them in moderation with attention to the calories if used in large amounts. If you want to use a salad dressing such as oil and vinegar it should be calculated as part of your fat calories. Mustard is better than ketchup (ketchup often has sugar) and mayo is rarely healthy. Spices are a great way to add flavor without calories; cinnamon, nutmeg, garlic powder, pepper, cumin, basil, cayenne, etc. Occasionally spices will add some health benefit.

8. Sugar-free beverages such as water, coffee, Crystal light, artificially sweetened waters, etc. are allowed ad lib. Black coffee is encouraged for its antioxidant benefits and mind/body boosting caffeine. Stay hydrated with at least an 8 oz glass of water with or after each meal.

9. Everyone should take a multivitamin, 2g of Omega-3 oils, Vitamin D 1000iu (if not in the multivitamin), and a probiotic supplement daily.

10. Time your meals such that a protein and carbohydrate meal follows your workout session within 1 hour. If you are in Muscle Building mode, have half of the meal before your workout session and the other half after. Those in Health Maintenance can have it either way, (after or split). Those in the fat burning category should keep the meal as a post-workout meal. Fat burners should skip carbohydrate in the post-workout meal and place it evenly in other meals or use its absence as part of their caloric deficit. By delaying the intake of carbs after a workout, you continue the fat burning potential of the workout for a few hours.

Yourgainplan.com can simplify this entire process by linking the numbers directly to your foods giving you per meal quantities and even a weekly shopping list. If you utilize this weekly it will help to adjust progress toward your goals. Using the website in combination with your information obtained by the *G.A.I.N.* Monitor will help you to see if your diet is in line with your activity and goals.

For the 3 goal categories there are also supplements that I encourage you to use in addition to those mentioned in #9 above.

1. **Health Maintenance:** This category is a baseline for anyone who wants to use supplements for improving longevity.

   - Polyphenol antioxidant: Resveratrol, grape seed extract, acai
   - Caffeine/Coffee
   - Arginine/Citrulline/Nitrates for healthy blood pressure
   - Creatine for vegetarians

   - CoEnzyme Q10, Niacin, Phytosterols

2. **Fat Burners:** This category needs to maintain muscle while mobilizing more fat and increasing fat burning.

   - Caffeine/Coffee
   - Green Tea Extract
   - Capsaicin
   - CLA

3. **Muscle Builders:** This category is goals to build muscle faster.
   - Whey Protein
   - Leucine/HMB
   - Creatine

Supplements

Guidelines for Choosing Supplements

1. **Use supplements that address deficiencies or goals in your training.**

   Deficiencies occur when your diet is lacking in important nutrients. If you know that you are not getting 5 servings of vegetables per day, you may be lacking in essential vitamins, minerals, antioxidants, and fiber.In this case you may need to consider a fiber supplement and a multivitamin. Similarly, you may be unable to sit down and eat 5 protein meals with lean meat, dairy, or eggs. In this case, you may find it difficult to get your protein requirements in and thus would benefit from a protein supplement. If you are a vegetarian, you may want to consider creatine and soy protein supplementation as your diet will likely be relatively deficient.

2. **Avoid taking "too much of a good thing", more isn't always better.**

   A very common mentality is that more is better. Just as we explained about over-training, you can over-supplement. Taking 500g of protein every day in the form of a whey protein drink is not going to turn you into the Incredible Hulk. Your body uses the protein it needs for building muscle and repairing your tissues and uses the rest as energy or just eliminates it by your kidneys. Excesses of protein to this extreme may even be detrimental to your physiology and result in organ damage. It is best to follow recommendations as given in this book or by reputable companies like GNC. Stimulants as found in fat burning and pre-workout supplements can be especially dangerous when taken in excessive amounts. There are many case reports in the medical literature and media that have enlightened the public of the possible harm of excessive use of stimulant supplements. This is not to say that you can't use these supplements, you have to use them as directed and in a sensible manner.

3. **Be scientific. Supplements may work for some and not others; figure out what works for you.**

I developed *The G.A.I.N. Plan* through a scientific perspective with the intention that you GAIN that same perspective. It is very important that you chose your supplements based on scientific evidence that they are actually worth your time. You should choose supplements that have been studied in subjects that are similar to you and prove effectiveness in your type of training goals. For instance, if you are well trained sprinter, a study that shows a supplement that improves sprint speed in otherwise sedentary persons may not apply well to you. If the study has not been done in an athlete such as yourself, you may need to conduct your own experiment. Even if there is an excellent randomized, placebo controlled trial that shows a supplement provides significant performance enhancement, this still doesn't mean that it will work for you! Thus, you should go about choosing your supplementation in a scientific way. You will be basically conducting a study where you are the only subject. The results will be anecdotal to everyone else and specific to you.

Pick a single supplement that is intended to help your specific goal.

The supplement may be a "proprietary blend" of multiple ingredients, but this type of study will only tell you that the blend does or doesn't work and not any one component of the supplement. For instance, you decide to take creatine monohydrate to improve your strength. However, you need to be more specific in your measured outcome. A specific hypothesis might be, "Creatine monohydrate supplementation will increase the number of dips I can perform in my first set of a workout" (It may be easier to determine the effects with an even more specific goal, such as increasing the poundage of your one rep bench press or bicep circumference measurements). Be sure to research the optimal dosage, timing of intake, and how long it usually takes for the supplement to take effect or is expected to last.

Perform baseline exercise and standardize conditions.

Perform a set of dips at the very start of a workout on a rested day before you start taking the supplement. Record the number of dips, time of day, and your diet over the last week.

You see, creatine is found in meat and if you had a lot of steak in the last week you may have a different response to creatine supplementation than a week where you had very little steak. Try to control your diet during your experimental period with the new supplement. If you aren't eating enough calories, or you aren't getting adequate protein, it is hard to gain strength and muscle even with added creatine.

Try to recreate the conditions and time of day when you return to do the dips after a course of creatine supplementation. Don't try to change more than one variable, such as multiple supplements or workout changes during the experiment time frame. Try to make the addition of the supplement the only change in your routine.

If you really want to take some bias out of your measurements, do this with a blinded, placebo control. This is a situation where you actually don't even know if you are taking the supplement or not. You need your friend, partner, or significant other to help you with this. Caution, if they aren't on the same page you might be annoying them. It works well if you have a supplement that you can mix into a protein drink. Creatine is often difficult to taste in a well-mixed protein shake. You can try a couple weeks of having a shake made by your helper where they either do or don't put the creatine in, but they don't tell you whether you're getting it or not.

Do the same challenge after supplementation in controlled conditions.

Do the same dip challenge before and after. Then, after a couple of weeks of no supplement/placebo (a wash out period), do it again with or without the creatine. Only your partner will know which you are getting. If you want to make it "double blind", you can have another person who doesn't know if you received the supplement or not count the number of reps that you were able to perform at each trial of dips.

Although this is a systematic approach to measuring the effects of a supplement, ther are a lot of variables that make it really difficult to know if the supplement tested really helped. As we have discussed previously, the placebo effect is very strong when doing a study on just you. The level of honesty with yourself must be held high Sometimes you just have to keep a log about how you feel, what your weight did, how your body fat percentage changed, and your consistency with taking the supplement. Real science done in a double-blinded placebo controlled randomized clinical trial of a supplement is the best way to know if a supplement might help you. Chances are that if you match the demographics and inclusion criteria used in the study, the results will apply to you.

If you want to research for studies on a particular supplement, search its name at www.pubmed.gov. Search the supplement name and what outcome you are interested in., i.e. Creatine and strength. If you are a student, chances are that you may have access to an online library where you can get articles of interest. While an undergrad, I would read about a supplement or training technique in a magazine, and I would look up the science in the library to find the scientific article it related to. By doing this I became scientific about my training and familiarized myself with the scientific process, thus improving my ability to critically analyze new products on the market.

4. **Beware of the Proprietary blends and rogue brands.**

Supplements aren't regulated by the FDA in the same way as prescription drugs. Although the FDA sets production standards and rules for making claims, they don't require clinical trials to prove quality, safety, or effectiveness Unfortunately, this often results in supplements on the market that can cause unforeseen harm. When enough harm is done, the FDA gets wind of the supplement and investigates it. If warranted they can then remove that supplement from the market.

The FDA doesn't require pre-market testing of dietary supplements. However, under the law, manufacturers are responsible for making sure their products are safe before they go to market. The claims on their labels must be accurate and truthful under the law. Even though dietary supplements are not reviewed by the government before they are marketed, the FDA has the responsibility to take action against any unsafe product that reaches the market. False and misleading claims made by supplement manufacturers can lead to legal action by the FDA and consumers who feel misled.

Stick with brands like the GNC brand that are known to have good production standards with regular testing of the quality and safety of their supplements.

5. **Check with your physician first.**
Dietary supplements do not come without risk. You are taking them to either make up for a deficiency, enhance your performance physiology, or improve your health. This means you are looking for an "effect". It almost goes without saying that anything that can have an effect on your body's physiology can have a "side-effect". That is, supplements and medications alike are not perfect and can

have additional effects that aren't intended or expected by the user. It is important to research the supplements you are taking to understand possible side effects.

This is especially a good idea for certain population groups. If you are pregnant, nursing a baby, or have a chronic medical condition, such as, diabetes, hypertension, heart disease, thin blood, anemia, or anxiety/depression be sure to consult your doctor taking any supplement. Parents should check with their pediatrician before giving any supplements to their child.

If you were prescribed a medication and you might have heard that a supplement could replace it, ask your doctor if they agree before you stop the medication. Supplements often contain active ingredients that have strong physiological effects that can interact with medications or medical conditions. Taking supplements with medications (prescription or OTC drugs) could produce adverse effects. Rarely the reaction of medication and supplements can result in life-threatening events. The most common example is for prescription blood thinners like Coumadin: ginkgo biloba (an herbal supplement for memory), aspirin, vitamin E, fish oil, can each thin the blood dangerously with Coumadin. Additionally, taking excessive vitamin K can counter-act the action of Coumadin.

It is especially important to inform your surgeon of any supplement you may be taking as many can affect healing or bleeding. Some of these supplements need to be stopped at least 2-3 weeks ahead of your procedure to avoid potentially dangerous outcomes.

Common supplements that can interfere with surgery:

1. Garlic
2. Ginger
3. Ginseng
4. Ginko
5. Feverfew
6. Bromelain
7. Licorice
8. Capsaicin
9. Saw Palmetto
10. Oil of Wintergreen (Methyl Salicylate)
11. Devil's Claw
12. High Dose Vitamin E

Dr. Prisk's Top 10 *G.A.I.N.* Supplements:

1. Multivitamin with Minerals

A multivitamin is probably the single most important supplement that all of us should take. It is fairly safe to say that most Americans do not consume enough of their daily vitamin and mineral requirements from the food we eat. I am not saying that a multivitamin should replace a healthy diet, but sometimes we skip on the veggies and fruits. To avoid deficiencies and any chance that these deficiencies reduce performance and recovery an inexpensive multivitamin is safe and effective. I recommend making a multivitamin with minerals part of your daily routine. Studies support that supplementation with a multivitamin may increase longevity in both men and women.

2. Whey Protein

As we have discussed earlier, whey protein is what I would call a very special protein from a health and muscle growth perspective. Our muscle has a relatively high proportion of branched-chain amino acids, and so does whey protein. The high leucine content of whey protein is thought to contribute to its better ability to rebuild muscle through activation of muscle protein synthesis. Whey protein isolates and hydrolysates are particularly useful. For men, consuming 30-40g within 1 hour prior to a workout and another 30g-40g within an hour post-workout is ideal. For women a dose of 20-30g before and after is probably enough to get your needed leucine. Whey protein shakes or bars can be used as a snack to meet protein requirements throughout the day. Microfiltered whey isolate mixes well in oatmeal and smoothies.

3. Fish Oil

Earlier we discussed the importance of omega-3 fatty acids and improving your omega-3 to omega-6 ratio. There are many studies to suggest that fish oil is effective at improving cardiovascular health and longevity. They may even improve recovery from exercise and its anti-inflammatory effect can sooth sore joints. Fish oil is a source of the best omega-3 fatty acids for your health DHA and EPA. Fish oil as a supplement or fatty fish is a better source of omega-3's than foods such as canola oil, soybeans, flax, walnuts and algae. It is important to note that if your diet is high in saturated fats and omega-6 fatty acid a supplement will have little effect on tipping the balance toward omega-3's. In combination with healthy fats in the diet, fish oil can be more effective in improving the balance. A dose of 2g per day of fish oil is most recommended.

4. Creatine

Creatine is perhaps the best performance enhancing supplements available to the strength athlete. If you are doing the Century Club Challenge creatine has the ability to improve your reps from a maximum of 10 to 11 in just one week of supplementation. The scientific literature supports it use and safety for a variety of sports and training conditions. Creatine monohydrate is the gold standard and has worked best for me. If you have stomach issues such as bloating or gas, PEG-Creatine [GNC Creatine 189] is much more tolerable and has better absorptive properties. Creatine is often loaded as 20g per day (4 doses of 5g) for 5 to 7 days and then maintained at 5 to 10g per day thereafter. Creatine is well absorbed as part of a post workout meal/shake. It can be safely taken continuously for 12 weeks. If you are involved in a sport that requires making weight, it may cause some water retention, so you may want to stop supplementation a week or so before your weigh-ins.

5. **Caffeine/Pre-workout**
Caffeine is another "ergogenic" supplement that can improve performance and recovery. It is so effective that it was once banned by the World Anti-Doping Agency (WADA) for use in competitions like the Olympics. At a dose of 3 to 9mg per kilogram caffeine has stimulating effects on central nervous system that improves focus and reduces perceived exertion. I recommend keeping your doses around 200-400mg per day as a pre-workout. This could be from simply drinking a 16 oz Starbucks coffee or from a pre-workout supplement. Black coffee has healthy effects in itself that could be beneficial to your health and longevity. I would caution you to keep this on the lower end until you get used to consuming that much caffeine. I would also recommend doses on the lower end as you get later in the afternoon. If you have caffeine after 5:00 PM, it may disrupt your ability to fall asleep. Doses greater than 600mg per day should be avoided for risk of toxic effects.

6. NO Boosters: Arginine/Citrulline/Nitrates

L-Arginine is an amino acid that not only works as a building block for proteins, it is also used in the synthesis of nitric oxide. Citrulline is a valuable precursor to arginine Nitrates are an excellent source of nitric oxide (as discussed earlier in the book). Nitric oxide is very important in many physiological processes. It is especially important in improving blood flow to various tissues. By supplementing with arginine and nitrates one can maximize the availability of nitric oxide. Arginine is often found in pre-workout supplements that are purported to boost nitric oxide (N.O.) and generate more of a "pump" by bringing more blood flow and nutrients to the muscle. Arginine can improve performance by reducing neuromuscular fatigue and potentially improve the anabolic response to exercise. It boosts collagen synthesis, improves wound healing, and boosts immune system function. Arginine is especially useful in recovery from wounds and injury as in surgery. Doses of 5g per day are typical for supplementation. I place all of my post-surgical patients on an arginine rich protein supplement.

7. Polyphenol Antioxidants

Antioxidants have effects that are very useful in recovery from exercise, especially after intense sessions that produce a lot of free-radicals. As we discussed earlier, free-radicals do have a valuable role in initiating pathways for adaptations to exercise. So, this is a

distinct case of where too much of a good thin
can hurt. However, the polyphenol
antioxidants are found in many of the foods
that *The G.A.I.N. Plan* find to be "super-foods"
and many people do not consume enough of
these foods. If your diet is lacking in
polyphenol rich foods, you will likely benefit
from their supplementation.

A polyphenol antioxidant is a type of
antioxidant containing a "polyphenolic
"or natural phenol structure. Plants make
these compounds as a natural defense against
the environment. For instance, grapes used
in wine making can be in harsh environments
that require great defenses against free-
radicals in their world. Thus, they produce
polyphenols like resveratrol (found in skins
of red grapes) as a defense mechanism to
boost their own longevity. Recent studies
suggest that resveratrol can activate anti-
ging proteins called sirtuins and limit
telomere shortening.

Oxidative stress and inflammation can reduce
performance and lead to fatigue after exercise.
If you are training with any level of intensity,
you will likely produce excessive inflammation
and oxidative stress. Using antioxidants
in moderation may help with your exercise
recovery and muscle soreness. Compounds
like resveratrol and grape seed extract are
excellent compounds for this purpose. The
doses of these compounds can vary greatly
so we recommend following the
manufacturer's suggested dosage (choose your
product wisely).

Antioxidants and Shocking the System

High intensity exercise produces molecules called free radical oxygen species or just "free radicals." Free radicals have gotten a bad name for themselves as they have been blamed for cellular damage leading to aging and cancers. Antioxidants, which are compounds which scavenge and eliminate free radicals, have flooded the supplement and food market. In fact, everything is marketed for having antioxidant properties including food and cosmetics. The problem is that there is a "Goldilocks" level for antioxidants vs. free radicals. Meaning, too little free radicals and you get no adaptive responses, but too much and you get cell and DNA damage. When we take excessive amounts of antioxidant supplements we can actually blunt that adaptive response and lose the benefits from our high intensity exercise. For those who don't get enough fruits and vegetables in their diets, I recommend antioxidant supplements in moderation for avoiding excessive free radical damage with intense training.

8. Melatonin

Melatonin 5mg per day improves sleep, adds antioxidant support, and boosts anabolic hormones. Melatonin was discussed in more detail in the sleep section.

9. **Vitamin D (Cholecalciferol)**

Vitamin D is structurally similar to steroids
such as testosterone but it is considered
a "secosteroid" because of differences in its
chemical structure. Vitamin D is formed in the
skin by a reaction of 7-dehydrocholesterol with
UV radiation from UVB light (sun or artificial).
It is converted to Vitamin D2 by the liver. It is
then converted to the active hormone Vitamin
D3 by hydroxylation in the kidneys.
In humans, Vitamin D affects skeletal muscle
cellularity, morphology, and ultrastructure.
It regulates the growth and development
of many different cell types, including those
of our interest, muscle cells. Studies have
shown that deficiencies of vitamin D or
lack of responsiveness to it because of genetic
defects, can cause atrophy of fast twitch type
II muscle fibers. The active form of vitamin
D functions via a nuclear receptor, much
the way anabolic steroids function, to stimulate
the expression of many genes related to
muscle growth and differentiation.
Recent scientific advances have identified that
vitamin D can also act through a non-genetic
rapid response stimulating muscle
development in cell cultures3.

In patients who have severe kidney disease,
a deficiency of the active form of vitamin D,
D3, had significantly lower measures of
physical performance and muscle size.
There are many studies that suggest
supplementation can improve muscle
performance and help prevent falls in vitamin
D deficient elderly patients. A recent meta-
analysis (review of many studies to combine

statistics) of seventeen trials revealed no significant effect of supplementation overall, but a significant improvement in strength was observed in the trials in which the mean starting blood level of vitamin D2 was 25 ng mL or below. The normal range is 40 to 80 ng/mL. Supplementation with daily doses of 800 to 1,000 IU consistently demonstrated beneficial effects on strength and balance in these elderly patients.

A great deal of research has been directed at correlating bone health with muscle health especially in our aging population. Deficiency of Vitamin D can result in significant muscle dysfunction and atrophy. Estimates of the prevalence of low vitamin D levels in US youth have ranged from 1% to 80%! Factors such as older age, winter season, higher body mass index, black race/ethnicity, and elevated parathyroid hormone concentrations

were associated with lower vitamin D concentrations in the blood. Levels tend to be more than 25% lower in the winter vs. summer months so bring on the sun.

Vitamin D is a good thing for bone and muscle, but you should limit your intake to 1000 IU twice per day unless otherwise prescribed by a physician for deficiency. Next time you are at your doctor's office, ask for a Vitamin D level as part of your labs.

10. **Pro-biotics/Pre-biotics**

The micro-organisms in our bellies are really just another organ system important for our health in too many ways to mention. They support the immune system, 80% of which is found in our GI tract. Taking pro-biotic supplements with viable health promoting microorganisms can improve digestive function, immune system function, and even sports performance. Pre-biotic supplements are those that promote healthy pro-biotic microorganism growth. These include fiber supplements and glutamine. The science behind intestinal micro-organisms is in its infancy and I expect great advances in the not so distant future. In the meantime, probiotic and prebiotic supplements to improve the microbiology of your gut is something I recommend. Greek yogurt and fermented foods are useful for boosting these healthy microorganisms but really supply limited concentrations of the organisms compared to supplements.

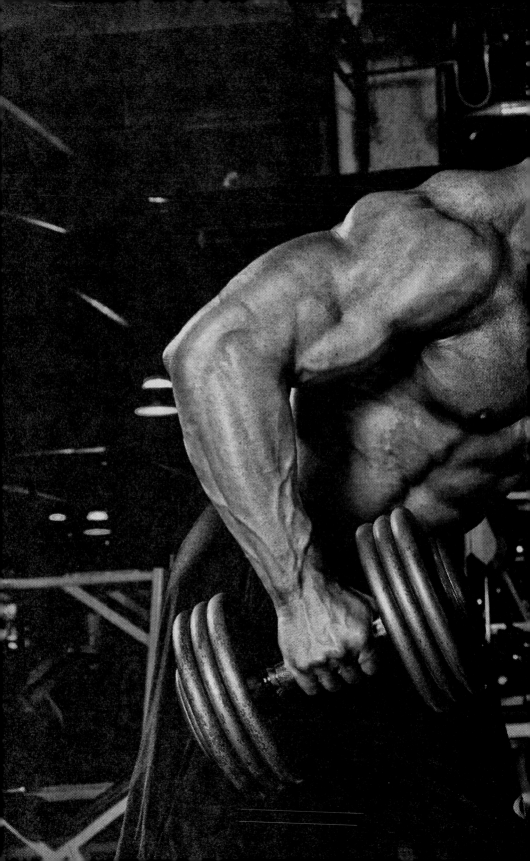

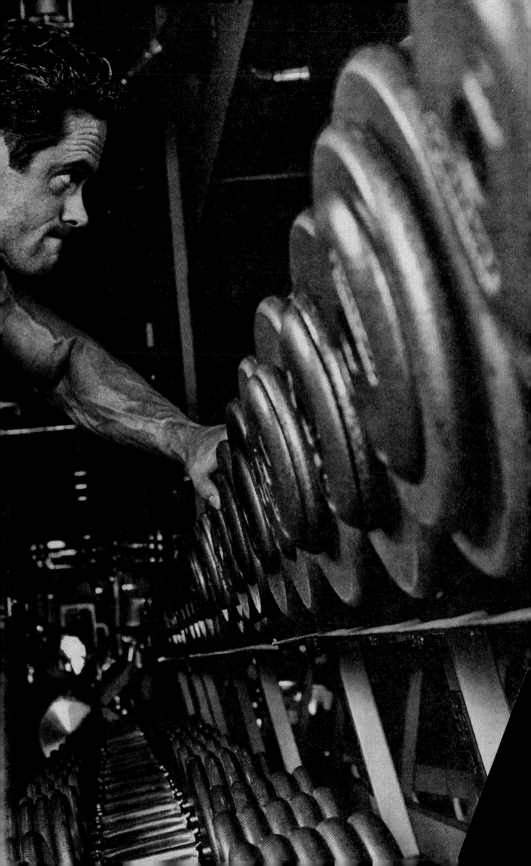

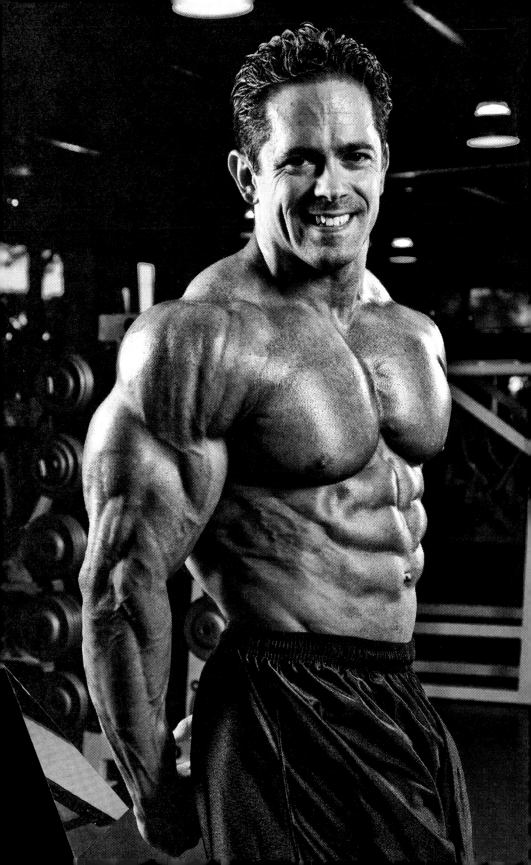

The Century Club Challenge

For those who are looking for a new challenge that goes beyond the usual lifting weights or cardio, I give you the Century Club Challenge. As I described earlier this is a series of exercises that I put together as a way to stay in shape after retiring from gymnastics competition. It gives a total body workout with variable levels of intensity to get a cardio and/or strength challenge.

The complete Century Club Challenge is meant to be something you train for as if you were doing a marathon. Although I can do this work out every other weekend, I have been doing it for 10 years. The "challenge" is to complete 100 repetitions of the 10 core exercises in less than 1 hour. In trying to complete this, you will find out what it means to be sore. You will also learn what over-reaching feels like. The day after doing the challenge, I tend to rest and recover eating plenty of protein, stretching, light cardio, and massage.

I am presenting you with the Century Club Challenge as a way to revive your competitive spirit. By challenging yourself and friends to this challenge you will reach new physical heights. You can create personal goals like finishing a ½ Century in 30 minutes or finishing 100 pushups in one set. You may just want to be able to perform 1 un-assisted chin up. No matter what level you start at there is a competition you can enter against yourself or your friends.

The Century Club Challenge embraces the concept of Performance As a Competitive Event (P.A.C.E.). First of all, you enhance your performance from workout to workout by competing with yesterday's self. Your goal is to gradually improve your performance on each exercise. This will culminate in completion of the complete challenge. Second, you can perform for others by showing off your ability to complete the exercises with proper technique and advanced techniques. You can share your originality in building upon the core exercises with variations that help those who are just starting or increase the intensity of the challenge. Finally, you can go to yourgainplan.com and join the leaderboard, post videos of your exercise variations, or challenge others to a contest. I encourage you to challenge others on Facebook, Twitter, and Instagram. Share in your success and failures. Use the support of your fellow challengers to overcome obstacles and learn new ways to recuperate.

Training for the Century Club Challenge will teach you about how your body works. It will help improve your strength, balance, endurance, and flexibility. With use of *The G.A.I.N. Plan* Monitor you will get in tune with your heart rate and use it to control the intensity of your training. By adjusting your workout to your heart rate you can decide on the heart rate training zone the meets your needs. If your goal is to get stronger, keep your heart rate below 65% of your HRmax with longer rest between sets. If your goal is to get a cardio challenge keep your heart rate over 65% for as long as possible. If you want a HIIT challenge shoot for >85% of your HRmax. Additionally, you will also learn how to pace yourself to accomplish the daunting task of completing the full challenge.

Use *The G.A.I.N. Plan* diet and supplement recommendations to boost your recovery and performance. Regularly adjust your diet to meet your macronutrient needs. Utilize stress relieving techniques and sleep better to recuperate faster. Objectively check your attitude, perceived exertion and performance in the gym. You have already learned to recognize the onset of nonfunctional over-reaching and OTS. Be a scientist, experiment and learn what works for you.

The Exercises

The core challenge includes the following 10 exercises:

1. Chin Ups/Pull Ups

2. Push Ups

3. Parallel Bar Dips

4. Handstand Pushups/Military Press

5. Barbell Curls

6. V-Ups

7. Back Extensions

8. Alternating Lunge Jumps

9. Squat Jumps

10. Single Leg Calf Rises

It is critical that you use strict form on each of the exercises. This is done by controlling your midsection with tight abdominal muscles. You should avoid swinging your arms or legs to finish reps. There shouldn't be any kicking or kipping on pull-ups or dips. You should have full range-of-motion with each movement. I recommend keeping the form of a gymnast with straight legs, pointed toes, and full extension

CENTURY
C L U B

See page 26 for photos of all Century Club Challenge exercises.

with each movement. If you have a tendency to kick or swing on hanging exercises try crossing your legs. On handstand pushups consider using a partner to balance rather than a wall; they will keep your legs together and tight.

Ways to Implement Century Club Workouts

Your body adapts to change and you grow from new experiences. Your mind and your muscles thrive on new experiences. When you try a new exercise for the first time, the next day you are often very sore. As your muscles recover from the soreness, they grow and adapt. Once they become accustomed to an exercise stimulus you need to change things up to stimulate further change. This can come in the form of changing the exercise itself in some small way or changing the resistance or intensity.

The simplest way to do the workout would be to complete 100 repetitions of each exercise in sequence. This doesn't mean that you have to hang from a bar until you complete 100 chin ups (if you can, you're elite already!), but the idea is to do as many as you can with each set until you reach 100 repetitions in the fastest time. The faster you try to finish the Century Club, the higher the intensity (don't neglet form). Doing all 100 repetitions at once is commendable but can be a little boring or for some, just impossible for others. I recommend changing up the workout and "shocking" the system regularly by doing a number of things:

Group Exercises

This involves making small circuits with a group of 2 to 4 exercises. For instance, take chins, dips, and pushups. Do 4 sets of 25 repetitions of each exercise; 5 sets of 20; or 10 sets of 10. You may find that one exercise is harder than the other, such as chins versus pushups. Most people can to more pushups in sequence than chin ups. In this case it may be worth using some assistance for your reps, such as a counter-balanced chin up machine or bungee cords. As your strength and endurance build, you can remove the assistance or even add weight (i.e. a weighted vest).

Also, you may want to mix in a midsection exercise (abdominal muscles) with the circuit to break up the pounding on the upper or lower body. For instance, combine chins, V-ups, and dips. This would allow your grip and upper body to relatively rest while doing the V-ups. You can also alternate between upper and lower body exercises.

Giant Circuits

One of the more challenging ways to get through this workout is to group all 10 exercises and do 10 to 25 repetitions of each for 10 to 4 times through the circuit, respectively. This method ensures that you hit each of the exercises at least once. If you are doing your 3rd time through the circuits and you find you've done enough you can stop and know you hit all of your body parts. You can push yourself through the challenge trying to complete each circuit in equal time and faster each visit to the gym. This can also be a method of learning to pace yourself; monitoring a constant heart rate and level of perceived exertion.

Alternating Upper and Lower Body

Another option is to move from an upper body exercise to a lower body exercise. For instance, one can go from chins to single leg calf raises to dips and then squat jumps, etc. This can effectively give the upper or lower half a little time to recover before the next exercise while keeping the heart rate up. One of the common effects of this sequence is that heart rate goes a little higher and blood shifts from top to bottom and vice versa which may be a little nauseating if you are unaccustomed.

Changing Body Positions

One of the nice things about the exercises in the CCC is that they can be performed in many variations of the core exercises. For instance, push-ups can be performed in various hand positions (wide, narrow, fingers in or out). Little changes in hand positions or body position bring into play different stabilizing muscles and thus brings in a new stimulus. I often perform my first 50 chin ups in an over-grip and then switch to pull-ups in an under-grip. Dips can be performed in an "L" body position, feet behind, or feet in front. Every exercise can be modified to change the muscle emphasis and intensity. You can change the positions from workout to workout or in working set to set. I would also encourage you to be creative in making your own variations and share them with the CCC community in the spirt of P.A.C.E.!

CCC and the Anaerobic-Aerobic Continuum

The CCC is a workout that combines anaerobic strength training with aerobic fitness. Each set that you perform in each of the 10 exercises is an anaerobic exercise. You can jump up and do chin-ups until complete exhaustion for a set and then rest until you are ready to perform more. For instance, I can jump up and do 40 chin-ups where it becomes very difficult to perform the last 5 reps and I can't hold on at the end. I would then jump down and rest until I can get back up and perform another 10 to 15. This would be largely anaerobic training.

The continuum comes into full effect when we focus on keeping our heart rate elevated with continuous movement. This can be done by doing a circuit of exercises that spare energy of other muscle groups. This would be like doing a circuit of chin-ups, v-ups, and squat jumps. Even though one muscle group like the arms gets tired with the first exercise, it recovers while you are doing another. However, your cardiovascular system is constantly pumping blood to other muscle groups and thus your heart rate and breathing rate increase. At this point you are entering a cardio training zone. If the exercises are done with too little rest or with too much intensity your body's need for oxygen might exceed the ability of your heart and lungs to deliver it. If this happens, you have exceeded a sustainable pace and you will have to rest and let your breathing and heart rate come down. Learning how to balance this oxygen exchange with exercise intensity is the key to P.A.C.E. and completing the CCC.

This is the same as if you were to start running a marathon at a 5 minute mile pace (essentially sprinting for me!). Your heart rate and breathing will cause you to stop well short of your goal. Alternatively, if you head out at a 15 minute mile pace, you may find this very boring with very little rise in heart rate or breathing. Learning what heart rate and exercise intensity is sustainable for you is part of the fun of training for a program like the CCC.

My Routine

I cycle my workouts doing the CCC workout every other Saturday. When training for a bodybuilding show, I do not perform the Century Club regularly, but I incorporate the core exercises into my split routine. I usually follow a workout split that looks something like what is written below.

Day 1. Back and Biceps; morning cardio

Day 2. Chest and Triceps; morning cardio

Day 3. Legs

Day 4. Shoulders, Abs, and Calves; morning cardio

Day 5. Rest. Stretch and massage.

Day 6. ½ to full Century Club Challenge (every other week) or weak body part

Day 7. Extra Stretching, massage, and low intensity cardio

When doing this training split I incorporate Century Club exercises into my body part routine. For example when training back I will warm up with 50 chin ups with various grips. When training chest I will finish my workout with dips and mix pushups in between exercise sets to keep the "pump" going. Occasionally, I'll start my bicep workout with a 100 rep set of barbell curls. Lunges and squats are essential components of any good leg training routine. V-ups and Back extensions are core exercises that can be done every other day.

The key to success in training for the Century Club Challenge is to listen to your body! If you are sore, work around the exercises that cause pain. Recover with adequate nutrition and rest. If you are stressed out, had very little sleep, or you are dealing with a nagging injury don't do the inciting portions of the CCC.

Workout Options

Another sequence that works well is as follows:

Day 1. Chins, Back extensions, bicep curls and cardio

Day 2. Squat jumps, Lunge Jumps, Single leg calf raises and high intensity cardio

Day 3. Pushups, Dips, Military press/handstand pushups and V-ups

Day 4. Rest; stretch, Massage

Day 5. Core strength, yoga/pilates, low intensity cardio

Day 6. ¼ to full CCC or Circuit training

Day 7. Rest; Stretch, Massage

For those who have only 3 days to train per week try to complete day 1, 2, and 3 with some cardio. It is also important to remember that if you get into a routine, morning fasting cardio can be done by just about anyone! Wake up before the kids and do 20 minutes of High Intensity Interval Training (will review in "G") , it will invigorate your body and mind for the coming day! Another way to approach the CCC is to use the exercises as a basis for your strength and conditioning throughout a stressful week. By completing one CCC over the course of 7 days you can be assured that you have strength trained your whole body even if it is in small segments at a time. Let's say you are stuck at the office every night working on a big project. Drop and do some pushups, v-ups, and lunge jumps to re-invigorate yourself. Record how many you do. If you squeeze in little circuits like this, you may be able to complete an entire CCC in one week. You may need to adapt some of your exercises using easily accessible *G.A.I.N. Plan* training gear (i.e. chin-ups and dips).

Using your markers of health provided by the *G.A.I.N.* Plan monitor, Your *G.A.I.N.* Planner diet log, and your *G.A.I.N.* Attitude assessment, along with assessing your joint/muscle soreness, you can determine when you are ready to push through a Century Club Challenge or any of its components. Be prepared to be sore the next day and plan to have a rest and stretch day possibly incorporating Yoga, Massage, and low intensity cardio after doing the challenge.

CCC Newbies

First, familiarize yourself with the exercises and determine which you can do and which you can't. If you can do 10 chin ups and 5 handstand pushups, then you are probable past the beginner level. Second, once you understand the exercises you can decide on the sequences and workout schedules. In this section we will give you a workout routine and schedule to try.

CCC Exercise Variations:

1.   Kneeling Pushups vs. Regular pushups

2.   Assisted Chin ups or bungee Lat pull downs vs. Chin ups/pullups

3.   Assisted Dips or bench dips vs. Dips

4. Barbell or bungee curls vs. 50lb bar

5. Dumbell or bungee military presses vs. handstand pushups

6. Simple crunches or tucked leg raises vs. V-ups

7. Superman back extensions/good mornings vs. hyperextensions

8. Standing lunges (+/- assist support) vs. lunge jumps

9. Air squats (+/- assist support) vs. squat jumps

10. Double limb calf raises vs. single leg calf raises

Start with a weekly routine that builds up your ability to master these exercises. Once you have mastered the lower level exercises start mixing in the more difficult versions of the exercises. For instance, try doing a few chin ups on your own and then do the rest with assistance.

12 Week Prep For Full CCC

This is a routine that can be done with variations in the exercises to increase or decrease the difficulty. It can be done with beginner level exercises or more advanced variations.

WEEK 1
(pace to HRmax of <75%):

Day 1. Exercises 1, 3, 5, 6. Perform a circuit of **10 reps**, 4x through then do 30min of LISS or 15min HIIT

Day 2. 2, 4, 7, 10 Perform a circuit of **10 reps**, 4x through

Day 3. Rest, stretch+/- LISS

Day 4. 6, 8, 9, 10 Perform a circuit of **10 reps**, 4x through then do 30min of LISS or 15min HIIT

Day 5. Rest, stretch +/- LISS

Day 6. 1x through 1-10 for **10 reps** each exercise x2 circuits; +/-20-30min of LISS

Day 7. Rest, stretch +/- LISS

WEEK 2
(pace HRmax of 75%-85%)

Same days, move faster with less rest, cardio

WEEK 3
(pace HRmax of <75%)

15 reps per set, 30min of LISS or 15min HIIT

WEEK 4
(pace HRmax 75-85% try to hit 90% HRmax in last circuit)

15 reps per set, 30min of LISS or 15min HIIT

WEEK 5
(pace HRmax <75%)

20 reps per set, 30min LISS or 15min HIIT; 1x through day 6 +10 rep 2nd circuit

---

WEEK 6
(pace HRmax <75%)

25 reps per set, 20min LISS or 10min HIIT; 1x through on day 6 [1/4 CCC]

WEEK 7
(pace HRmax 75-85% try to hit 90% HRmax in last circuit)

25 reps per set, 20min LISS only; 1x through on day 6 [1/4 CCC]

WEEK 8
(pace HRmax <75%)

25 reps per set, 20min LISS or 10 min HIIT; do 2nd 10 rep circuit day 6 [1/4 CCC +1/10th]

WEEK 9
(pace HRmax 75-85% try to hit 90% HRmax during last circuit)

25 reps per set; **20min LISS only**; do **2nd 10 rep** circuit day 6 [1/4CCC +1/10th]

WEEK 10
(pace HRmax <75%)

25 reps per set; **20min LISS or 10min HIIT**; do **2nd 25 rep** circuit day 6 [1/2 CCC]

WEEK 11
(pace HRmax <75%)

25 reps per set; add 10 rep 5th set; **10min HIIT**; do **3rd 10 rep** circuit day 6 [1/2 CCC +1/10th]

WEEK 12
(pace HRmax 75-85% try to hit 90% HRmax during last circuit)

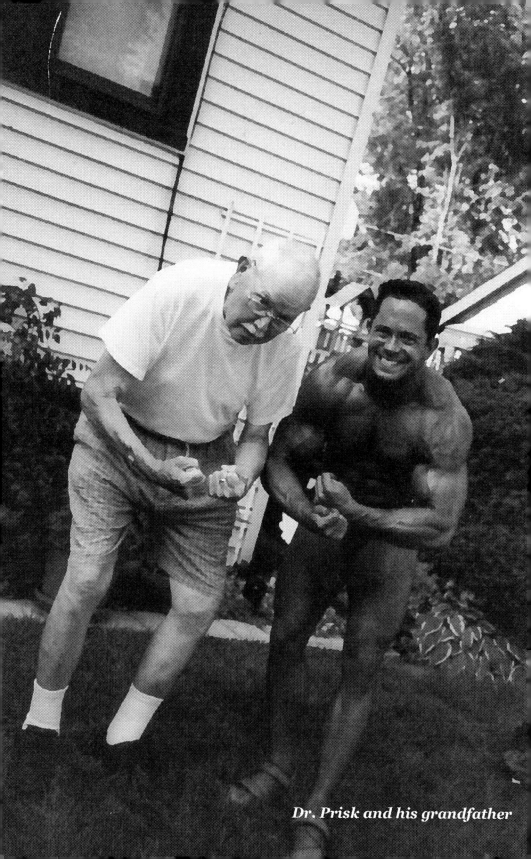

Dr. Prisk and his grandfather

Who Is Dr. Prisk?

Dr. Victor Prisk is a nationally recognized board certified orthopaedic surgeon who had fairly humble beginnings. Dr. Prisk was born and raised in the western suburbs of Chicago to a hard working family of a beautician and a telephone-pole climbing repairman. His beginnings were rich in adversity and contributed to his recognition of life challenges.

He was born a twin with his brother Anthony Prisk. The birth would present the first challenge in his life, as his mother was ill with a life-threatening disease called fatty liver of 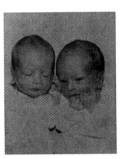 pregnancy. Without an emergency C-section the mother and babies would certainly perish. The twin babies, although a month premature, survived the ordeal without physical harm. Unfortunately, Dr. Prisk's mother lost her life that day. Undoubtedly it was a sad day for the Prisk family. They would recover as the boys would grow up with their sisters to be healthy and successful.

Dr. Prisk and his twin competed in soccer, T-ball, and played musical instruments in their youth. They were very competitive with each other. They would push each other through fierce competition to be their best at whatever they attempted. Their competitive nature led to great accomplishments. They would go their separate ways with Tony becoming a world champion trumpet soloist and symphonic musician in the Philadelphia Orchestra.

Chapter 6

Victor the Gymnast

Being a small freshman in high school, Victor found the sport of gymnastics appealing for the strength that it displayed. His world for the next 4 years would revolve around gymnastics. The still rings event was his first love. Two things about the rings interested to him; one, the strength it displayed and two, despite a lack of experience or talent, hard work on the rings produced visible results.

To advance his skills in the gym, Victor became a student of the sport and eventually a coach.

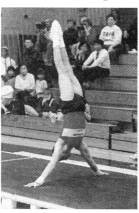 As his skills improved he would coach kids and share his love for the sport with his younger teammates. In order to improve his performance, he began reading fitness magazines. In particular, *Muscular Development* and *Muscle & Fitness* contained science based articles that immediately grabbed his attention. The magazines would fuel his interest in medicine.

However, another life changing moment occurred during his sophomore year of high school. While on his favorite event, he generated too much swing on the "still" rings and accidentally flew off the rings during a gymnastics competition. He would land missing the mat and injuring his ankle. The next day, he had his first visit of many with an orthopaedic surgeon. The doctor would make an indelible 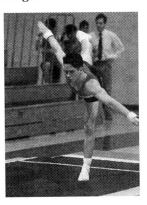 impression on this young athlete. Upon leaving that first office visit he would give his mother a self-fulfilling prophecy that he would become an orthopaedic surgeon. But, driven to be the best he would return to be conference all-around champion that season.

Victor would recover from his ankle injury, subsequent knee surgery, broken hand, and hernia repair in his junior year to become a regional and sectional gymnastics champion. His injuries fueled his desire to become a surgeon and sparked his interest in the sciences.

On the side, he had a keen interest in flying airplanes. He had been a member of the Civil Air Patrol, and found the movie *Top Gun* quite inspiring. In his senior year of high school an opportunity to apply to the United States Air Force Academy arose from his relationship with University of Illinois gymnastics coach C.J. Johnson. Victor succeeded in acquiring a congressional appointment to the Academy. The next stage in his life was set.

Victor attended the Academy, but encountered the most difficult decision of his life to date after basic training. Unfortunately, during basic training he ended up with a bad case of bronchitis that put him on bed-rest for the first 2 weeks of his first college semester as a 4th class cadet. This led to a great deal of harassment by senior cadets and the stress led to weight loss, loss of strength, and academic challenges. He made the difficult decision to transfer to a traditional university, knowing that the transition would be filled with uncertainty.

As luck would have it, the Academy coach, Lou Burkle was friends with the Iowa State University gymnastics coach Dave Mickelson (now a coach at AFA). Iowa State had an open scholarship and it was offered to Victor. He would jump on the opportunity as working in a warehouse and coaching gymnastics to 6 year olds was wearing on his patience in the transition.

Victor would learn valuable lessons about his body while at Iowa State. Coach Michelson was quick to realize that his persistent shoulder problems were a consequence of over-training. With the mentality of "more is better" Victor was naïve to his vulnerability for injury and Coach Michelson opened his eyes to this. He rotated his training and rest (periodization) making him an event specialist limiting him to his 4 best events,

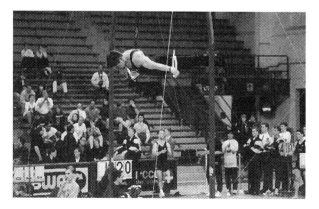

high-bar, rings, parallel bars, and vault. After
a rough freshman year, Victor would qualify to
the NCAA Championships in his sophomore
year. Unfortunately, he would be the last male
gymnast to compete for Iowa State on the rings.
At the end of his sophomore year, the Men's
Gymnastics team was discontinued at Iowa State.
He decided to stay at Iowa State and pursue
research opportunities, the Honors College,
tutoring, and Tae Kwon Do. However, his love
for gymnastics was quite pervasive and he
would soon return to the sport with renewed
motivation. Going into his senior year, he built a
small ring tower with rings 2 feet off the ground
in his dorm room. He would train strength moves
on this tower and drive 5 ½ hours to Chicago

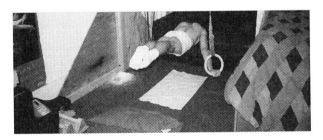

from Ames on the weekends to train with Mark
Diab of Premier Gymnastics. Mark was a 2
time former NCAA National Ring Champion
and helped Victor to master the rings. With the
goal to compete in the Windy City Collegiate
Invitational, he trained intensely in the months
leading to this competition, developing original
skills to impress the judges.

At the 1996 Windy City Invitational he would
catch the eye of the judges and former Iowa
State gymnast and Michigan State University
head coach Rick Atkinson. After weeks of

discussion and communication with the NCAA it was determined that Victor was still eligible to compete in his 5th year of college.With a scholarship in hand to be a ring specialist, Victor would make one of the easiest decisions of his life and apply to graduate school at Michigan State.

As a graduate student in the department of physiology Victor did lab research on diabetes, worked with the Bayer Corporation, and studied for the medical college admissions test (MCAT). With an atypical schedule, he trained late in the afternoon even after much of the gymnastics team had already called it a night. He would have a relatively injury free season and attained a 1st place ranking on the still rings during the 1997 season. After becoming an NCAA All-American with a second place finish at the National Championships

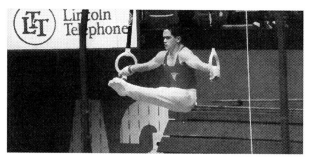

his competitive drive led him to continue to shoot for first place through medical school.

Dr. Prisk the Medical Scholar and Dancer

In June of 1997, Victor received the phone call which would make his dream to be an orthopaedic surgeon a reality. He was accepted to the University of Illinois, College of Medicine at Chicago. He would become first year class president, pursue research in cardiovascular physiology, and excel in academics. Although he continued to train gymnastics with C.J. Johnson at the university he looked for other outlets of stress that arose from the rigors of medical school.

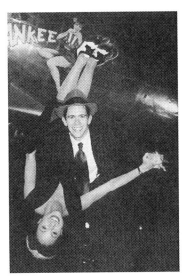

Underlying his interest in gymnastics was also an interest in dance. He had been an avid hip hop dancer in high school and minored in dance at Iowa State. In fact, he participated in shows for the Iowa State auditioned dance society, Orchesis. He would find interest in the fad of swing dancing that was taking the Windy City by storm in 1998. After only of few months of lessons and intense practice he formed a performance dance troupe called *Hep Cat Swing* with his dance partner and 2 other couples. They would perform all over the city and eventually the country, until the national infatuation with swing died down. It would provide a much needed release from the stress of medical school. You may ask how he was able to do this in medical school? With the guidance of a close friend, Cardiologist Dr. Ross Vandorpe, he had taken many of his medical sciences such as gross anatomy, biochemistry, pharmacology, and microbiology as an undergraduate and graduate student.

Although he had interest in medical specialties like urology, cardiology, and even psychiatry, his passion for orthopaedics prevailed in his senior year. After graduating at the top of his class with high honors, Dr. Prisk would move to the University of Pittsburgh for his orthopaedic surgery residency training. The university had a strong reputation in research and sports medicine which was quite attractive to Dr. Prisk. Although he was skeptical of moving from Chicago to Pittsburgh, the steel city would steal his heart from day one and he resides there to this day.

Dr. Prisk never did things the easy way as you might have guessed. He did the extended 6 year residency with an added year of research. He chose Pitt Ortho because of muscle injury and stem cell research being performed by Dr. Johnny Huard. After a year in the lab, which also allowed him to continue to pursue dance and gymnastics, he came to another turning point. Gymnastics was taking a toll on his shoulders and despite desires to pursue a qualification to the world championship team an injury would end that dream (Birth of *G.A.I.N.*).

After residency, Dr. Prisk took a fellowship in foot and ankle surgery with an emphasis in dance medicine and reconstructive surgery. The ankle injury from high school went full circle as he looked to care for those athletes he could relate to most. Under the guidance of Dr. William Hamilton at the Hospital for Special Surgery of the Weill Cornell Medical College in New York City he would participate in the care of the *New York City Ballet* and *The American Ballet Theatre*. An invaluable experience that gave him the ability to recognize the unique problems associated with the intense training involved in professional dance. He also performed and published basic science research on ligament injuries in the ankle (J Bone Joint Surg Am. 2010 Oct 20;92(14):2375-86).

Dr. Prisk the Bodybuilder

Dr. Prisk recalled his fitness magazines from high school and the bodybuilding competitions. Here was a sport that combined his interests in exercise physiology, sports nutrition, working out with weights, cardiovascular exercise, and stage choreography into one discipline where he could still utilize gymnastics skills and perform.

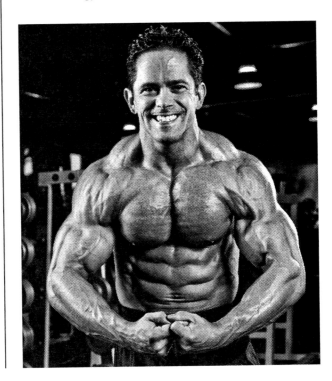

After encouragement from the President of the International Federation of Body Building and the National Physique Committee, Jim Manion, Dr. Prisk returned to Pittsburgh as an Assistant Professor of orthopaedic surgery at the University of Pittsburgh. While at the University, Dr. Prisk cared for Pitt Athletics and the *Pittsburgh Ballet Theatre*. He has currently taken this experience and his research to help in development of a new healthcare system in Pittsburgh, including his Institute for Performance Medicine with the Allegheny Health Network. He lives in the Pittsburgh suburbs with his wife, Dr. Kristina Curci. He married a psychiatrist who also shares his interest in bodybuilding and sports nutrition. Through training together they were both able to become national champions in the sport of bodybuilding. They enjoy traveling together and playing with their puppies, Louie and Lucy.

These experiences have molded Dr. Prisk's expertise and led to the development of *The G.A.I.N. Plan*. As you read through this book you will find examples of how his experiences have shaped this plan. You may have had experiences similar to these that led to your own stories. Feel free to share your story at www.yourgainplan.com.